COPING WITH CEREBRAL PALSY
Answers to Questions Parents Often Ask

Michael A. Horvat

COPING WITH CEREBRAL PALSY

Answers to Questions Parents Often Ask

by
Jay Schleichkorn, Ph.D.
School of Allied Health Professions
State University of New York at Stony Brook

University Park Press
Baltimore

UNIVERSITY PARK PRESS
International Publishers in Science, Medicine, and Education
300 North Charles Street
Baltimore, Maryland 21201

Copyright © 1983 by University Park Press

Composed by University Park Press, Typesetting Division

Manufactured in the United States of America by
The Maple Press Company

Library of Congress Cataloging in Publication Data
Schleichkorn, Jay.
Coping with cerebral palsy.

1. Cerebral palsied children.   2. Cerebral palsy.
I. Title.   [DNLM: 1. Cerebral palsy.   WS 342 S341c]
RJ496.C4S348   1983   616.8'36   82-17339
ISBN 0-8391-1768-X

Table of Contents

Foreword

Over the last several years, medical technology has virtually created a revolution in care of the high risk mother and infant. Significant reduction in infant mortality has clearly resulted. Morbidity, especially in relation to neurological deficit, also appears to be less, particularly for babies of near normal birthweight. For the very small infants, survival is now the rule; but it seems that they will more likely have significant developmental deficits such as cerebral palsy, and possibly more extensive and severe involvement. Thus, the future trends suggest increasing severity of the condition, though perhaps an overall reduction in those affected.

This situation is of major importance for the primary medical practitioner who must increasingly take responsibility for early identification and referral of children who may have developmental problems. The practitioner must assess the needs of both the child and family, see that the child has an appropriate evaluation or referral for more extensive workup, and must help the family locate services for ongoing therapy and management.

Many physicians themselves have little sophistication in these areas and would benefit from additional training to better meet these responsibilities. An area of special need is providing understandable background information to the family of a child diagnosed as having cerebral palsy.

Families faced with such a diagnosis often have had months to years of confusion and uncertainty about the child's limited progress. They often have been bombarded by "advice" and well-meaning "assistance" by friends and relatives that frequently further cloud or confuse the picture of what is wrong and what needs to be done. Up to the present time there has been very little written material to which the family can turn for assistance and information. Even the well-meaning and sympathetic physician who wishes to enlighten those affected has not had good reading resources to recommend.

This situation will now be remedied to a considerable extent with the publication of *Coping with Cerebral Palsy: Answers to Questions Parents Often Ask,* by Jay Schleichkorn. This work is based on material obtained from parents of children with cerebral palsy through the use of a questionnaire and interviews. It represents in retrospect those areas of concern about which information and guidance was felt to be needed and which would enable a much better adjustment in dealing with present and future problems of the child.

At last the physician has a solid source of reference for families to help them make the adjustment to caring for and understanding the needs of the child with cerebral palsy. It is hoped that the medical profession will take full advantage of this source and utilize it fully. Similarly, therapists, social workers, teachers and others dealing with the child with cerebral palsy should use the work extensively with families with which they come into contact.

Alfred L. Scherzer, Ed.D., M.D.
Clinical Professor of Pediatrics
Cornell University Medical College
New York City, New York

Preface

A phone conversation with a parent many years ago left me with a lasting impression and a deep concern for parents of children with cerebral palsy. After his child was seen in a major diagnostic center in New York City, a father called me and during the conversation said, "Now that I know my child has cerebral palsy, do I feed him...DO I FEED HIM?" Obviously, no one spent any amount of time talking with this distressed parent. He indicated that the physician seemed to be in a rush, the social worker had several people sitting in the waiting room—no one was able to tell this distraught father how to handle his disabled infant.

All of the plans for raising a healthy, normal child may be shattered when parents are told, "Your child has cerebral palsy." The future of the child is immediately placed in jeopardy. Parents face confusion and a long-term struggle. Hundreds of questions come up which cannot be answered immediately or to the satisfaction of the parents. Professionals who are available may discuss cerebral palsy using medical terms that are not completely understood by all parents. Some parents turn away from professionals, families, and friends to face their problems alone. Other parents seek information from those parents who may also have a child with cerebral palsy.

In my thirty years of experience working with families of children and adults with cerebral palsy, I have found a common denominator among all parents. They constantly seek answers to many questions in order to better understand the total ramifications of the condition known as "cerebral palsy."

Perhaps there were attempts to answer the questions by many different professional personnel, but the parents were unable to assimilate all of the information, did not interpret what was heard, or would not accept what was said. Parents have also indicated that professionals are not always consistent in their responses to questions.

I have been encouraged by many parents and professionals to prepare a publication that would attempt to answer most of the questions parents raise when coping with a child with cerebral palsy. Through my work and involvement with parents over many years, I have heard hundreds of questions and shared their concerns. In 1980, as part of a doctoral study, I completed a survey on the informational needs of parents of children and adults with cerebral palsy. The study involved 193 families. More questions were added to my collection. Professional personnel have also given me input as to the type of questions parents ask most often. Every question represents a matter of great importance to the parents and must be addressed.

In this publication, the questions are answered based on available information, through searching the literature, talking with professional personnel, meeting with parents and adults with cerebral palsy, and my own experience. It must be emphasized that it is possible to write pages and pages in answering many of the questions. Brevity does not infer that a question is unimportant. Where necessary, I have attempted to keep medical jargon and technical terms at a minimum. Certain medical terminology is used and parents should become familiar with those terms. Knowing the language will bring about better communication between parents and professionals.

Should the parents want further information, the references and recommended readings suggest where it can be found. Probably the best resources for more material would be through the services extended by a public library, medical facilities, or those professional personnel working with your child.

Readers will also note there is quite a lot of information about the adult with cerebral palsy. Many parents of children beyond the infant years have expressed the need for information about the problems faced by those with cerebral palsy in adulthood.

I recognize that every person with cerebral palsy represents a unique individual. No ready answers will fit every situation. However, by sharing the concerns of other families, the family faced with the daily problems of their child will be better informed and capable of meeting the challenge of coping with cerebral palsy.

This publication, together with appropriate support from within the family, parent groups, various organizations, and professional personnel, all involved in the total care and management of children and adults with cerebral palsy, may hopefully serve those parents who at one time or another may have asked the question, "DO I FEED HIM?"

Acknowledgments

The preparation of this publication is the result of the involvement of many people who unselfishly gave of their time in reviewing material, responding to certain questions, and offering me advice, guidance, encouragement and support.

My appreciation is extended to the following:

— the members of my Doctoral Committee from The Union for Experimenting Colleges and Universities, Dr. Frank Reissman, Dr. Mary Sheerin, Dr. Barbara Baskin, Dr. Jane Porcino, Dr. Irving Bialer, and Dr. Albert Curtis

— Marilyn Rauth, Director of Educational Issues Department, American Federation of Teachers, Washington, D.C., for use of her material in responding to questions related to education

— Sal Gullo of the United Cerebral Palsy Association of Nassau County and Joan Malden of Associated Therapies, for giving me access to parents of children with cerebral palsy

— Virginia Browning and Susan Hayes, New York Chapter, American Physical Therapy Association, for sharing the Glossary of Terms

— Mr. and Mrs. Charles Bull, Mr. and Mrs. Thomas Hackett, Mrs. Martin Eaton, Dr. Leonard Silverstein, Dr. Paul Jordan, Dr. Isabel Robinault and Mrs. Margaret Schilling for reviewing material

— Dr. Alfred Scherzer for his criticism and most valued comments

— Dr. Leon Sternfeld of United Cerebral Palsy Associations for his initial encouragement

— the faculty of the Physical Therapy Department, School of Allied Health Professions, State University of New York at Stony Brook for their constant support: Michael Helland, Clifton S. Mereday, Marian Pernetti, Janice Sniffen, Barbara Silvestri and Sharon Waldman

— the staff of the Health Sciences Center Library, Stony Brook for their assistance in my continued search for material

— Gloria Mitchell, the physical therapy department secretary, for assistance in typing much of the material and watching my grammar

— Dr. Edmund McTernan, Dr. Walter Heimer, Dr. Eleanor Schetlin, Dr. Isabel Robinault, Dr. and Mrs. Robert Craig, Robert O. Hawkins, Una Haynes, and Elaine Becker, and my three sons, Raymond, Peter, and Henry, all of whom made me realize that the project could be completed

— my dear wife, Marianne, who allowed me to spend countless hours reviewing material, reading books, attending conferences, and sitting at my typewriter, knowing that it was all going to be most worthwhile

— the staff at University Park Press, editors David P. Miller, and Maureen McNeill

— to all those parents of children and adults with cerebral palsy who participated in my original survey and offered questions

To all, accept my deep appreciation!

to
Leonard, Naomi, Philip, Larry, John,
Clara, Norma, Susan, Anna, Veronica,
Jill, Barbara, Judy, Linda, Douglas,
Isabelle Ann, Arthur, Neil, Faith, Alfred,
Ruth, Kenneth, Nancy, George, Karen,
Muriel, Jimmy, Paul, Pat, Gil, Fran,
Annabelle, Tom, Ernie, Ida, Richard,
Eddie . . . . and the many other children
and adults with cerebral palsy who
have been so much a part of my life.

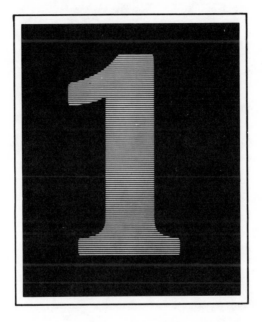

CEREBRAL PALSY
The Condition Itself

WHAT IS CEREBRAL PALSY?

Cerebral palsy is a complex condition and an umbrella term often used to cover a variety of problems related to birth injury.

The term *cerebral palsy* may refer to different neurological conditions that produce a disability because of the muscular incoordination and weakness.

Cerebral palsy may also be referred to as a *developmental disability,* a *neuro-motor dysfunction,* or a *developmental motor disability.*

Reading the literature, one can find several different definitions. Cerebral palsy is defined as a group of disorders of movement and posture due to a defect or lesion of the immature brain (Bax, 1964).

Cerebral palsy is a chronic disability characterized by aberrant control of movement or posture, appearing early in life and not the result of recognized progressive disease (Ellenberg and Nelson, 1981).

The American Academy for Cerebral Palsy and Developmental Medicine defines cerebral palsy as a persistent, but not unchanging, disorder of movement and posture appearing in the early years of life and due to a traumatic or inflammatory brain damage or again to a nonprogressive disorder of the brain, the result of interference during development.

How Many Children with Cerebral Palsy Are Born Every Year?

Estimates vary on how many children are born with cerebral palsy because it takes months and even years before a true diagnosis is determined. A major problem arises from the use of different terminology and methods of diagnosis.

It has been estimated that one in every 200 to 300 babies born in the United States will have cerebral palsy, which means there will be approximately 25,000 new cases each year (Heppenstall and Centerwall, 1977).

Another researcher points out that there was a time in 1950 when between 25,000 and 30,000 babies were born with cerebral palsy, but since then the number has declined to 12,000 to 15,000 due to increasingly widespread application of preventative measures (Goldenson, 1978).

The United Cerebral Palsy Research and Educational Foundation report, '"Doubling the Odds Against Cerebral Palsy," indicates that the number of infants born with this condition in 1978 was under 10,000—less than half of the comparable number for 1958.

More recent studies and review of the occurrence of cerebral palsy in industrialized countries concludes that the evidence did not support the notion of a steady decline in cerebral palsy. Reports of cerebral palsy prevalence rates per live births in recent decades in western nations show a mixed pattern (Kiely et al., 1981). Some countries showed a decline, others showed a rise, and some remained stable.

The incidence of cerebral palsy has been documented in various studies around the world, and the rate varies from 1 to 5.9 per 1,000 (live births), depending more upon the variety of methods used for identification than actual incidence (Thompson and O'Quinn, 1979).

How Many People with Cerebral Palsy Are There in the United States?

With the variety of problems related to cerebral palsy and the condition often being classified as *developmental disability,* obtaining an accurate figure of the total population of people with cerebral palsy continues to be difficult.

The United Cerebral Palsy Association, the major national voluntary agency serving those with cerebral palsy, estimates that there are one-half million persons with cerebral palsy in this country.

Why Me?

This is a question that is asked by many parents over and over again. Because cerebral palsy has no respect for any nationality, race, color, creed, or economic status, it can occur in any family.

There is no answer to this question.

Did I Personally Do Something to Cause Cerebral Palsy in My Child?

It would be inconceivable to suggest that a mother would purposely take any action to have a child with cerebral palsy.

Despite paying close attention to suggestions made by the physician and having good obstetrical care, cerebral palsy does occur.

Parents who interpret that having a child with cerebral palsy is their fault for some action taken in their lives will spend more time seeking reasons and will have less energy to meet the needs of the family. Should either or both parents feel that there is some type of blame or guilt, professional counsel and advice should be sought.

Is Cerebral Palsy Inherited?

It must be emphasized that cerebral palsy is the result of some type of damage to a part of the brain. Parents of a child with cerebral palsy should not look to hereditary factors as the reason for the damage. Clear-cut cases of cerebral palsy of genetic (chromosomal) abnormality are rare (Cruickshank, 1976).

If parents have heard that there is a hereditary link to cerebral palsy, it may be because of a secondary condition. If, as an example, diabetes is inherited and the diabetic condition disturbs the development of the fetus, one may say that there was some type of hereditary connection. Only because of this fact has it been estimated that at least 10%

of cerebral palsy may have some origin in hereditary factors. Overall, the influence of such factors requires further study and what is presently known is not completely clear.

Is Cerebral Palsy a Disease?

A disease is often defined as any departure from health, or an illness in general. When one speaks of a disease, it may bring to mind a specific cause and a destructive process in an organ or a contagious condition. Such is *not* the case with cerebral palsy.

Crothers and Paine (1959) made the point by stating that "the term cerebral palsy does not designate a disease in any usual medical sense. It is, however, a useful administrative term which covers individuals who are handicapped by motor disorders which are due to non-progressive abnormalities of the brain."

Why Is Cerebral Palsy Occasionally Referred to As *Little's Disease*?

In the late 1800s, the term *Little's Disease* was primarily applied to what we call cerebral palsy.

William John Little, a physician in London, in 1861 reported his study of 63 patients whom he followed after birth. His paper, "On the Influence of Abnormal Parturition, Difficult Labours, Premature Birth, and Asphyxia Neonatorum, on the Mental and Physical Condition of the Child, Especially in Relation to Deformities," was published as part of the transactions of the Obstetrical Society of London in 1862. The paper became a classic in describing the connection between birth histories and children with brain damage.

In Little's time, he became well known for his work in orthopedics and the term *Little's Disease* was applied to many conditions related to congenital muscular paralysis.

Literature today, in describing the early history of cerebral palsy, will often refer to the outstanding contribution made by Dr. Little.

Does Cerebral Palsy Affect Boys More Than Girls?

The incidence of cerebral palsy appears to be slightly higher in boys than in girls: a ratio of 1.4 boys to 1 girl has been reported (Gilroy and Meyer, 1979).

What Signs Can Parents Look For That May Lead to the Suspicion of Cerebral Palsy?

If for some reason your pediatrician has not recognized the possibility of your child having cerebral palsy, there are important growth and developmental landmarks that parents may notice. Understanding normal growth and development would be helpful to all parents.

When parents have other children, the first person to notice that something is not right with the new baby may be the mother. It may be observed that the baby does not suck properly or swallow well. There may be an unusual stiffness to the infant's arms and legs, especially noticeable when changing diapers. Constant irritability, poor sleep habits, no reaction to sudden movements or loud noises, or an overall floppiness will lead the parents to believe something is wrong. Suspicions may be further aroused if there was a history of problems during the pregnancy which gave cause for the child's being considered a high-risk infant. Very often, the child's grandparents will observe some small difference in this child that is not apparent in their other grandchildren. It is often very difficult for grandparents to tell this to their children, but experience is on their side, and their observations may be very worthwhile.

As soon as the parents become aware of a problem, the physician should be called, and the child should be seen for an extensive examination. It may be only slow development or a lag in maturation, but until the parents can be certain, there will be many hours of anxiety.

When Should a Diagnosis of Cerebral Palsy Be Made?

Diagnosis will depend on many factors. Although it is hoped that a diagnosis can be made in infancy, a single examination is not sufficient. Considering the high-risk factors or difficulties at delivery, together with a history and knowledge of neurological signs, the physician may have good reason to consider a diagnosis of cerebral palsy or some other neurological condition.

It has been reported that it may take 2 years to determine if a high-risk infant has a developmental disability or is completely normal. A major study reported that 98% of the children with cerebral palsy were diagnosed by 48 months of age (Barsch, 1968). In another study, it was found that 96% of the children with cerebral palsy were diagnosed by 48 months (Schleichkorn, 1980). Actually, in both studies the majority of the children were diagnosed by the age of 2 years.

It is important that the parents do not pressure the physician or the evaluation team for a diagnosis. Many of the developmental signs must be observed before a definite answer can be given to the question, "Is there something wrong with my child?" At the same time, while waiting for the diagnosis or some conclusion to the many observations by professional personnel, the parents will need ongoing support.

Years ago, many parents reported that their physician stated, "Your child will grow out of it." Despite all of the advances made in the practice of health care and the amount of knowledge available about cerebral palsy, it still is possible to hear such a misstatement.

The important point for parents to remember is that there is no great rush or vital need to have a diagnosis. Knowing that there is some kind of problem and delayed development, parents can still initiate a plan of action.

TYPES OF CEREBRAL PALSY

What Parts of the Brain Are Damaged in Different Types of Cerebral Palsy?

The brain is a very complex organ. It is obvious that there are many areas that can be damaged. That is one of the major reasons it can be said that no two persons with cerebral palsy are the same.

To simplify the geography of the brain, many publications refer to three major areas in which damage results in the more typical types of cerebral palsy.

Generally, damage to the motor cortex or cerebrum leads to spasticity. The cerebrum is the largest part of the brain consisting of two hemispheres. The cerebrum is concerned with sensations and all voluntary muscular activities.

Athetosis, recognized by involuntary, uncontrolled movements, is the result of damage to the area in the midbrain known as the basal ganglia. It is composed of four masses of gray matter located deep in the cerebral hemispheres.

Impairment of the cerebellum, located in the rear of the skull, results in loss of balance and incoordination. The ataxic classification goes with damage in the cerebellum.

What Is Spasticity?

The person with cerebral palsy who falls into the *spastic* category demonstrates a hyperirritability of the muscles to stimuli. The muscles tend to tighten up, which may lead to contractures and deformities.

Spasticity results from damage to that part of the brain known as the cerebrum.

Spasticity should not be confused with paralysis. The child will still have voluntary movement, but it will be slow and "jerky" at times. Often, tightness prevents the child from functioning in a normal manner. Parts of the body most likely affected are the wrists, elbows, hips, knees, and ankles.

Those persons with spastic paralysis may also demonstrate other problems, such as sensory loss in the hands, perceptual difficulties, and seizures, in addition to the contractures in the various muscle groups.

A recent study involving a review of available information on patients in the St. Louis area indicated that there has been a notable increase in number of cases in the spastic group (O'Reilly and Walentynowicz, 1981).

How Do You Describe Ataxia?

Damage to that area of the brain known as the cerebellum results in the type of cerebral palsy known as ataxia.

The most distinguishing characteristic of the child or adult with ataxia is the inability to maintain balance. It is difficult to identify ataxia in an infant until the child starts to walk. About 2% of persons with cerebral palsy fall into this classification.

What Is Athetosis?

Athetosis is a major classification of cerebral palsy. Persons with athetosis may also be classified as having dyskinesia (literally translated as having difficulty with movement). The child or adult with athetosis may have facial grimaces and some drooling, as well as slow, irregular, twisting, uncoordinated movements. Speech is often involved, due to the difficulty the child has in controlling muscles that are required to produce speech. Hearing may also be affected.

The child with athetosis probably suffered damage to the area of the brain known as the basal ganglia. The athetoid form of cerebral palsy is not frequently seen before 18 months of age as its appearance depends upon the development of major motor patterns and brain maturation (Scherzer, 1974).

Recent writings in the medical literature indicate a decline in the number of cases of athetoid cerebral palsy seems to have been established in many parts of the industrialized world (Paneth et al., 1981).

Referring again to the St. Louis area study (O'Reilly and Walentynowicz, 1981), the diagnostic category of athetosis showed a dramatic decrease in number of cases.

Is Athetosis a Coordination Problem Related to Cerebral Palsy?

Because athetosis is directly related to involuntary movements, it becomes obvious that any attempt to perform fine movements will result in uncoordination.

When a child with athetosis attempts to reach for a glass or pick up a pencil, the condition may prevent the child from making the simple movement and the child will appear to be uncoordinated. The amount of movement may vary from time to time.

It must be stressed that the child is not clumsy . . . he or she just cannot control the movement. This must be taken into account in all activities. Large gross movements will present less of a problem.

Is It Possible to Have Both Spasticity and Athetosis?

A "mixed type" of cerebral palsy has been identified in cases in which the child exhibits characteristics of spasticity and athetosis. It appears that athetoid persons are most likely to have some form of spasticity, whereas the child who has been diagnosed as pure spastic has some involuntary movements.

In mixed types, usually the lower extremities are spastic and the upper extremities (hands and arms) are involved with the athetoid movements.

Does the Child Have Athetoid Movements When Sleeping?

It is generally accepted that the child with athetosis does not have the involuntary movements during sleep. Movement apparently stops when the child is in a sleeping posture, secure and comfortable.

Parents will notice that movement will occur when the child is disturbed in bed when being tucked in the blanket or if the bed is moved. Loud, sudden sounds may also initiate movement during sleep.

Can a Baby with a Flaccid Form of Cerebral Palsy Become Spastic?

Flaccidity refers to a softness, a limp-like condition which, when applied to muscles, means there is a lack of tone or *hypotonia*.

Flaccidity of muscle tone is usually a temporary or a passing condition in cerebral palsy. It may be seen in early infancy and eventually is followed by more of the characteristics of spasticity or the athetoid type of cerebral palsy (Bobath, 1966).

CLASSIFICATIONS ACCORDING TO SEVERITY

What Classifications Are Used to Determine Severity of the Child's Condition?

Basically, the degree of severity is derived from describing what the child with cerebral palsy needs to perform in the activities required for daily living. Rusk (1977) described the classification of severity as follows:

Mild   The patient needs no treatment, because he has no speech problems, is able to care for his daily needs, and ambulates without the aid of any appliances.

Moderate   The patient needs treatment, because he is inadequate in self-care, ambulation, or speech. Braces and self-help appliances are needed.

Severe   The patient needs treatment, but the degree of involvement is so severe that prognosis for self-care, ambulation, and speech is poor.

Has the Infant Mortality Rate in the United States Changed in the Past Decade?

In 1960, the overall infant mortality rate in the United States was 26 per 1,000 live births. By 1975, the rate was down to 16.1. In 1977, data indicates the rate was 14.5 per 1,000 live births (Richmond, 1978).

There is now confirmation that the infant mortality rate in the United States reached a new low in 1980, 12.5 infant deaths per 1,000 live births (Wegman, 1981) (see Figure 1).

What Is the Mortality Rate of Children with Cerebral Palsy?

There seems to be a mortality rate of approximately 10% within the first 5 years of life for children with cerebral palsy (Warfel and Schlagenhauff, 1980).

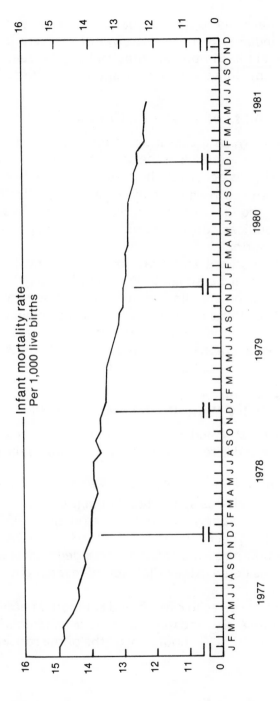

Figure 1.   Trend in rates for successive 12-month periods with each month indicated. (Source: U.S. Department of Health and Human Services, Public Health Service, Office of Health Research, Statistics, and Technology. 1981. Monthly Vital Statistics Report, Vol. 30 No. 6 September 15, p. 3)

It has also been reported that, because of better obstetric and pediatric care, the survival of the very low birthweight infant has improved, thus making the quality of life for surviving infants an important issue (Driscoll et al., 1982).

Will My Child Eventually Be Normal?

Cerebral palsy, as a condition, is incurable. It is also considered nonprogressive in the sense that, once the damage to the brain has occurred, the condition is established.

The degrees in which cerebral palsy shows itself, from a very minor condition to a completely severe physical and mental handicap, do not permit the parents to think in terms of "normalcy."

A child whose legs may be severely involved most likely will never be a marathon runner but may be able to demonstrate outstanding abilities in other areas of endeavor. The efforts of many professional disciplines, working closely with the parents of children with cerebral palsy, are directed at emphasizing those abilities. Parents must be hopeful at all times, but also realistic.

Are Most Children and Adults with Cerebral Palsy Mentally Retarded As Well?

You will probably find a different figure referring to mental retardation and cerebral palsy in every major publication on the subject.

When cerebral palsy first became a familiar term in the United States, it was suggested that approximately 70% of the children had normal intelligence (Phelps, 1950). More recently, it has been reported that at least half of the persons with cerebral palsy are mentally retarded, although most may be considered in the mildly retarded range (Goldenson, 1978).

Using IQ scores to classify and categorize people is still quite controversial, and many parents of children with cerebral palsy feel that IQ should not be the prime consideration in determining intelligence. It does require a variety of tests.

It has also been reported that a large number of children with cerebral palsy have specific learning disabilities. What one must recognize is that all too often the associated problems of cerebral palsy give an outward appearance of retardation based on how people and our society stereotype others. Such problems may include poor speech, drooling, incoordination, peculiar gait, and poor posture.

Even the most severely physically handicapped person with cerebral palsy (and there are many) may have escaped damage to that part of the brain involved with intelligence. A careful assessment and evaluation by a professional team will be the major factor in determining to what extent the child is or is not retarded. If it is determined that the child is retarded, the parents must be concerned with obtaining appropriate services and training to meet the needs of the child.

Is Mental Retardation a Direct Result of Cerebral Palsy?

The answer to this question is similar to "which came first... the chicken or the egg?"

Many publications indicate mental retardation can occur as a result of over 200 causes. It is also generally recognized that mental retardation is related to a problem that may occur before, during, or after birth. There are also people with mental retardation for whom no specific causes for the condition can be found. Similar situations arise in cerebral palsy. It, too, is known to occur before, during, or after birth. There are hundreds of possible problems that may result in damage to the brain which in turn may be classified as cerebral palsy.

The fact that there is brain damage affecting motor control distinguishes cerebral palsy from what is typically considered to be mental retardation. Certainly, whatever the cause of cerebral palsy may be in a specific child, there remains a concern that retardation may also be present.

Multiply handicapped persons may be epileptic, deaf, blind, and cerebral palsied and still not be shown to be retarded. It all depends upon the location of the damage to the brain.

Parents should recognize that there are similarities in causes of cerebral palsy and mental retardation, but one does not necessarily accompany the other.

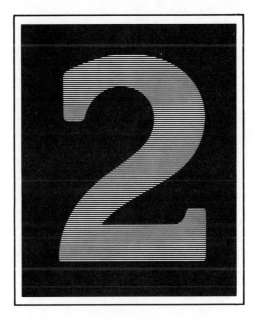

CAUSES OF
CEREBRAL PALSY

MAJOR CATEGORIES

What Are the Causes of Cerebral Palsy?

Generally, the causes of cerebral palsy are grouped into three major categories according to the period in which the potential problem may develop. Some examples of causes are listed.

Prenatal   From the time of conception to the time of labor, any one of the following may occur.

Anoxia: due to some problem with the umbilical cord
Maternal infection: due to a viral or infectious agent such as rubella, toxoplasmosis, herpes simplex
Metabolic disease: diabetes, heart condition, hyperthyroidism, severe asthma
Rh factor: Rh sensitization

Natal   From the onset of labor to the actual birth of the baby, any one of the following may occur.

Anoxia: due to some obstruction involving the cord
Asphyxia: resulting from a mechanical respiratory obstruction
Analgesics: administering of drugs affecting the respiratory center of the infant
Trauma: any injury to the baby's head during labor, hemorrhage, forceps application, poor position of the infant
Pressure changes: too fast a delivery, too slow a delivery, Caesarean section
Prematurity: complications at birth, respiratory distress, "small-for-date" babies

Postnatal   From the time of and after the birth of the child, any one of the following may occur.

Trauma: damage to the head by fracture or wounds
Infections: childhood fevers, meningitis, encephalitis, brain abscess

Vascular problems: hemorrhage, thrombosis
Anoxia: strangulation, carbon monoxide poisoning
Neoplasms: tumors, cysts, hydrocephalus

There are all types of complications that can occur. It would be important to parents of children with cerebral palsy to have some knowledge about possible problems, especially in anticipation of having more children. A planned discussion with appropriate professional personnel is in order.

PREMATURITY

How Is Prematurity Related to Cerebral Palsy?

Prematurity has been defined as the state of an infant born any time before completion of the 37th week of gestation or born with a birthweight of 2,500 grams (5.5 pounds) or less.

The literature today refers to prematurity based on both the weight of the baby and the length of gestation. It is clear that prematurity (referring to low birthweight) is the most common single associated factor in cerebral palsy. A number of studies have shown that as many as 39% of children with cerebral palsy have a history of low birthweight (Scherzer and Mike, 1974).

How Many Premature Babies Are Born Every Year in the United States?

The rate of prematurity has not changed significantly over the past 25 years. The rate according to the United Cerebral Palsy's Research and Educational Foundation appears to be about 8.5% of the newborn population each year. This means a quarter of a million babies are born prematurely every year (Sternfeld, 1978).

Are Most Premature Babies Likely to Have Major Problems?

In a major study completed in 1958, at least two-thirds of infants in the low birthweight group had some kind of physical, mental, or emotional problems in their infancy and childhood.

More recently, in a review of 1,503 cases of patients with cerebral palsy, it was reported that prematurity was the most common etiological factor, occurring as the primary factor in 341 cases or 22.7% (O'Reilly and Walentynowicz, 1981).

If a child is born prematurely, however, this does not automatically indicate that a serious impairment will result.

Have Chances for Survival of Premature Babies Improved?

Babies born in the late 1940s and early 1950s of low birth-weight (under 3½ to 4 pounds) had a significant chance of having problems related to cerebral palsy. Those babies born in the 1960s and 1970s had a much better chance for survival. Some of the factors suggested that brought about the more favorable results include regionalization of care, good transportation to centers where prenatal monitoring and postnatal intensive care are available from skilled people all of the time, and improved nursing care (Avery, 1978).

Recent studies demonstrate that many of the newborn infants with problems are being saved due to the neonatal intensive care programs. As these infants are saved, however, a modest increase in the prevalence of disabling conditions may also be seen (Paneth et al., 1981).

What Is Being Done to Prevent Prematurity As a Cause of Cerebral Palsy?

Studies are being conducted through medical centers to reduce the rate of prematurity and its effect on the central nervous system.

Federal funding through the National Institutes of Child Health and Human Development (NICHD) allows for research in the problems of pregnancy, infancy, and developmental disabilities. Prevention of cerebral palsy, prevention of prematurity, and efforts to minimize respiratory distress are examples of NICHD activities.

Major foundations and voluntary health organizations such as the United Cerebral Palsy Associations Research and Educational Foundation and the Easter Seal Society, currently support research projects that complement NICHD's efforts and further the investigation of prevention of cerebral palsy.

In addition, the development of special services in hospital centers with neonatal and special newborn facilities offer intensive care to the premature infant.

How Can Pediatricians Be Helpful in Diagnosing Cerebral Palsy in Premature Babies and at Younger Ages?

The pediatrician can be most helpful in assessing the child's development in conjunction with the total history of the pregnancy and birth. Usually, it is the pediatrician who gives the first thorough physical examination to the newborn infant.

As the child is seen by the pediatrician, all aspects of growth and development will be checked. Patterns of movement go hand-in-hand with the maturation of the brain. The pediatrician's awareness of prematurity as one of the major causes of neurological impairment or cerebral palsy may add to the suspicion of a problem. Until all factors are considered, a diagnosis may only be tentative. There is no rush to giving a label to the child or making a definite diagnosis.

A program of early intervention is still indicated for the benefit of the child even before a conclusive diagnosis is made.

Is the Infant Who Is Born Prematurely and Placed in an Incubator Because of the Need for Oxygen a Sure Candidate for Brain Damage?

It is known that the administration of oxygen, which saves the lives of numerous premature and low birthweight infants, also causes the development of retrolental fibroplasia. This is a condition in which an opaque fibrous membrane develops on the posterior surface of the eye lens. In many instances this leads to permanent blindness.

The occurrence of the condition was noted in the early 1950s, when studies showed the possible connection between oxygen therapy in premature infants and permanent damage to the eyes.

Today, there are recommendations on the use of oxygen established by medical authorities that have reduced the problem (James and Lanman, 1976). When oxygen is required to maintain life of the high-risk infant, careful control of the oxygen input, length of time in the incubator, and observation should eliminate this concern for premature babies.

Can Breech Delivery Result in Cerebral Palsy?

In a breech delivery, the buttocks or leg, instead of the head of the infant, comes out first. Approximately 3% of all labors result in such delivery.

The possibility of brain damage occurring during a breech presentation is increased due to anoxia (oxygen deficiency). Because of this, and with the ability to determine the position of the baby, the physician may recommend the Caesarean procedure.

The St. Louis area study of 1,503 patients with cerebral palsy (O'Reilly and Walentynowicz, 1981) included almost 3% (43 cases) due to breech delivery.

If the Baby Must Be Delivered by Forceps, Will There Be Brain Injury?

Use of forceps is often a common procedure when assistance is required in delivery to prevent prolonged labor. However, there are some common forceps delivery injuries that may result. There could be facial paralysis when the facial nerve is compressed resulting in a temporary paralysis of the muscles near the mouth. Recovery is usually complete.

Forceps delivery could result in pressure marks appearing near the scalp. These too, tend to disappear after awhile.

A hematoma (or swelling, or mass of blood) is often seen 6 to 8 hours after delivery. No treatment is required.

Mothers often claim that the child with cerebral palsy was damaged by the obstetrician using forceps. Handled properly, the forceps are a major factor in assisting the fetus to make an entrance into the world. The skillful obstetrician will make the decision when to use forceps.

Handled improperly, the forceps may cause permanent damage involving injury to the eyes or nose, severe shoulder problems, and even fracture of the skull.

After Having a Child with Cerebral Palsy, Can a Mother Have a Second Child with Similar Problems?

No one can tell a mother of a child with cerebral palsy that there is an absolute guarantee that future pregnancies will result in a perfectly normal child. The pregnancy and birth process is just too complicated.

When one looks at the mother who presents no risk in having a child, the good health of the mother seems to be the vital factor. Various studies have been reported indicating that the mother who has a history of problems, such as delivering a stillborn or a premature infant, or early bleeding, will be more likely to have continued problems. The physician of your choice should be able to determine what chances the mother has of repeating problems at birth. Many parents of children with cerebral palsy do have additional children who are normal. There are also those (a rare occurrence) who occasionally have a second child with some type of developmental disability.

In a study and follow up done in Israel (Margulec et al., 1966) of 560 families with children with cerebral palsy, 34 families were found to have had at least two children with cerebral palsy.

With good counseling and advice from professional personnel, the parents must make the determination about having more children.

PREVENTION

Is There Any Preventive Medicine or Action Parents Can Take Against Cerebral Palsy?

Yes—good prenatal care is most important! Expectant parents should be prepared to be involved with good medical supervision as early as possible during the pregnancy. Very often, the mother may not be aware of her pregnancy until the second or third month. During that time, the fetus has developed rapidly and could have been subject to many different possible problems. It is, therefore, vital that if there is any possibility of a pregnancy, the mother should be cautious about exposing the fetus to damage. Much has been written about such exposure to smoking, drugs, radiation, alcohol, and other factors. Involvement in situations in which the mother may be exposed to infectious diseases should be avoided.

There is no "spoonful of medicine" that taken during pregnancy will prevent cerebral palsy. Good common sense applied to the total health of the mother is important. Regular checkups with your physician will give the parents the opportunity to discuss the developing fetus and any problems that may arise.

Can German Measles (Rubella) Cause Cerebral Palsy?

German measles, or Rubella, is generally a very mild disease. In children, the disease may cause a rash, some swelling of the glands in the back of the neck, and a slight fever. Although it is not dangerous to children, exposure to women who may be pregnant is cause for concern. This is especially true for those women who work in settings with small children or who have school-age children of their own who may be exposed to the disease at school.

German measles can be harmful to the developing fetus in the mother's womb. The earlier in her pregnancy an expectant mother contracts the disease, the greater danger to her child. German measles is known to cause major problems, such as mental retardation, cerebral palsy, hearing loss, visual problems, or combinations of these.

A United Nations health publication (1976) describes the seriousness of German measles, especially around the eighth or ninth week of pregnancy. At that time, it may produce hearing defects in babies of 12% to 30% of such mothers exposed to the disease.

It is imperative that every child be protected from German measles. In the long run, this would prevent the disease from spreading and causing untold damage to newborns. An innoculation is available and every child should be innoculated at approximately 15 months of age.

What Is the Rh Factor?

The Rh factor was first recognized in experimental work done with the Rhesus monkey. The factor is part of the blood. Most people have it and are called Rh + (positive). Those who do not have the factor are called Rh − (negative). Whether you have positive or negative Rh does not make any difference to your health. However, when a Rh − woman marries a Rh + man, her children may be subject to Rh disease, which can damage the fetus before or soon after birth. Rh disease can be prevented by knowing what factor is present.

Of special concern is the birth of a second child, because the mother may become sensitized by the first child if the first child was Rh + .

How Does Rh Disease Actually Occur?

When a baby inherits Rh positive blood from the father and the mother has Rh negative blood, the mother's body may develop substances that can harm the baby during pregnancy. This rarely happens with the first baby, but the danger increases with each pregnancy.

If the fetus is Rh + , Rh antibodies produced in the mother's blood may cross the placenta and destroy fetal cells. Such destruction may result in a child being born with mental retardation, anemia, heart defects, or other birth defects such as cerebral palsy.

Rh disease can be prevented. A new serum is available (RhoGAM) that, when injected into the Rh negative mother within 72 hours after the birth or miscarriage of each Rh + child, protects the next Rh + child she may have. The serum does not work for the woman who has had a child with Rh disease because the harmful substances have already developed in her·blood. Future babies of these mothers can be treated with blood transfusions given to the baby either before or just after birth.

It is very important that parents know their blood type and Rh factor. This should be checked with your doctor and involves a simple blood test.

Would a Caesarean Delivery Prevent Damage to the Baby?

It is well known that there are advantages and disadvantages to having a baby by Caesarean delivery. It has been suggested that the baby should not be subjected to any possible problems with delivery through the vaginal canal, when the potential for a problem can be effectively avoided through a Caesarean.

It would be difficult to prepare a list of every possible indication for a Caesarean section because of the number of combinations and complications that could develop. Primarily, the need for the procedure may be due to a problem with the fetal heartbeat, abnormal posture of the fetus, anticipated breech delivery, irregular labor, and related situations.

Like any operation, a Caesarean presents a danger to the mother as well as the child. A study completed in Europe indicated Caesarean section carried a maternal death rate ten times higher than other forms of delivery. An analysis of a group of women who died in association with Caesarean section showed that disease of the mother was the main cause of death (Stembera, Anamenacek, and Polacek, 1976).

Would a Caesarean section prevent damage to the baby? The most important advantage is that such delivery may improve the baby's chance of survival and reduce the likelihood of learning disabilities, mental retardation, brain damage, or certain physical handicaps (Donovan, 1978).

Are More Babies Being Delivered by Caesarean Section Today Than in the Past?

The rate of births by Caesarean section has almost tripled in the last 20 years for the United States as a whole, now accounting for approximately 17% of all births.

There are specific medical indications for a Caesarean section. A 1979 Department of Health, Education and Welfare report, however, in describing the main reasons physicians gave for the rising number of Caesareans, stated that they feared the "threat of a malpractice suit if a Caesarean section was not performed and the outcome was 'less than a perfect child'" (Seliger, 1981).

Should I Have Undergone the Amniocentesis Procedure to Determine If My Child Had Cerebral Palsy?

Amniocentesis is a procedure in which the amniotic sac is punctured by using a needle and syringe to remove some amniotic fluid. The material is then studied to determine if there is a potential for a known hereditary disorder or for conditions related to maternal age when the mother is over age 40.

Such fetal abnormalities usually detected through the procedure include hereditary problems such as hemophilia, recessive genes for sickle cell anemia, and neural tube defects. Because cerebral palsy is not included in such hereditary conditions, it is questionable whether amniocentesis could have forewarned the parents that there would be brain damage.

How Safe Is the Amniocentesis Procedure?

There is controversy about the complete safety of the procedure.

A report of 3,000 cases from the University of California at San Francisco supports the conclusion that the procedure is relatively safe. In another situation, however, a report on amniocentesis to the Medical Research Council of the British Royal College concludes that the added risk of the procedure indicates it is not to be regarded as fully safe.

The British study was based on 2,500 cases compared to matched controls who did not have amniocentesis. The study showed that there was only slight risk to the mother but an increased risk of fetal loss of 10 to 15 in a thousand with a similar increase in certain types of major infant morbidity.

The British report recommends that amniocentesis be carried out only in instances of serious concern for fetal risk (Kaiser, 1979).

If I Had Been Attached to a Fetal Monitor, Could the Damage to My Child Have Been Prevented?

The purpose of monitoring is to detect and display the fetal heartbeat. It allows for continued assessment of the baby's progress.

The use of the electronic fetal monitor (EFM) was once reserved for only 5% to 10% of all high-risk pregnancies. With its more frequent use, the physician should be able to determine if the fetus is in any type of distress.

According to the Center for Disease Control in Atlanta, there has never been any controlled study demonstrating that EFM produces healthier babies. In fact, studies have shown it does not make any difference (Seliger, 1981).

Considering the possibility that use of the EFM may indicate the fetus is in trouble, it does become another tool for the obstetrician to use in assisting with the delivery. Any damage that may be seen at birth could have happened in spite of the monitoring process. Normal labor and delivery involves a great deal of stress, and it is traumatic for both the baby and the mother.

Further investigation will have to take place to determine whether actual monitoring in all cases of pregnancy will prevent damage to all babies.

Is the Lamaze Method of Delivery As Safe As People Say?

Ask mothers about their delivery by the Lamaze method, and they probably will tell you it is the only way to have a baby. The method should be safe as long as the mother has not been placed in a high-risk category and no problems are anticipated at delivery.

Although it may be difficult to compare various types of delivery methods, a major study to determine whether Lamaze childbirth preparation is harmful or beneficial was undertaken between 1975 and 1976 at Evanston Hospital in Illinois.

The study involved 2,051 patients, 500 of whom chose the Lamaze method of prepared childbirth. Using matched controls (age, race, parity, and educational levels), the data suggests that the Lamaze method is beneficial in many ways.

The Lamaze-prepared patients had only one-fourth the number of Caesarean sections and one-fifth incidence of fetal distress. The perinatal mortality of the Lamaze patients was one-fourth that of the controls, and post-partum (after childbirth) infection was one-third of the controls. The Lamaze group had fewer perineal lacerations.

The control patients had almost three times as many cases of toxemia (distribution throughout the body of poisonous products of bacteria) of pregnancy and twice as many of prematurity as the Lamaze-prepared patients (Hughey, McElin and Young, 1978).

In an editorial comment about the study, appearing in the June 1978 issue of the Obstetric and Gynecology Journal, Dr. John W. Greene, Jr. makes reference to the difficulty in assessing some of the general statements often made about the benefits of the Lamaze method, such as "maternal satisfaction, better babies, healthier babies, and happier mothers with smoother convalescence." Referring to the study, Dr. Greene states, "However, this study does show statistically significant benefits to Lamaze-prepared patients: a lower rate of Caesarean section, less toxemia, a lower incidence of prematurity, less fetal distress, and a lower incidence of both maternal morbidity (rate of disease) and the use of antibiotics."

No doubt many more studies will be undertaken with patients involved in various natural birth preparations. Long-range follow-up studies will also be important to determine the outcome of the deliveries and whether or not there is a marked reduction in brain-damaged children attributable to Lamaze preparation.

EARLY RECOGNITION

Why Isn't Cerebral Palsy Recognized at Birth?

In most situations, cerebral palsy may be recognized at birth or at least the possibility of some type of brain damage may be suspected. This is especially so if there were high-risk factors involved in the development of the fetus or major problems during the delivery.

Actually, an infant with brain damage may not show immediate signs of any problems. As the infant matures and the damaged brain does not allow for normal development, the concern for cerebral palsy may be more evident.

There are particular signs that parents may note that would lead them to be suspicious of any problems. These signs may include the infant's poor response to the sucking reflex, jaundice or yellowing of the skin, convulsions, unusually strong reactions to noise, stiffness, and constant irritability.

The pediatrician, in examining the infant after delivery, should be aware of any complications that may have developed and be able to alert the parents to potential problems.

This is another reason why good postnatal care is important for the baby and the parents.

How Many Children with Cerebral Palsy Are One of Twins?

Throughout several texts on cerebral palsy, reference is made to the additional high risks in twin births. Although premature birth is characteristic of multiple births, studies indicate that prematurity alone cannot be considered the cause for one of the infants having cerebral palsy.

The second born of the twins seems to be more frequently at high risk. This may be due to lack of oxygen at delivery or some other form of chronic distress.

As to numbers of twins being born with cerebral palsy, several studies have been reported. In 1953, at the Lenox Hill Pre-School Cerebral Palsy Clinic in New York, among 100 cases selected at random, physicians found "six representatives of pairs of twins, as compared to the general incidence of one pair of twins in 85 deliveries (Cardwell, 1956).

An extensive study in Israel of a large population of persons with cerebral palsy included 551 single births and 21 born as one of twins. Based on the known information from this study, it would indicate that less than 4% of that sample population came from multiple deliveries (Margulec, 1966).

O'Reilly and Walentynowicz (1981), in their study of etiological factors involving 1,503 patients with cerebral palsy, reported that 5% of the cases involved twins. Of the twin births in the study, 41.5% were premature.

Why Are There Still So Many Infants Being Born with Cerebral Palsy?

The causes of cerebral palsy are so varied that it is most likely cerebral palsy as a condition may never be totally eliminated.

Leading researchers and authorities in the field of cerebral palsy predict a reduction of 50% or more in the occurrence of cerebral palsy will be achieved within this century. In the last decade, the incidence of cerebral palsy in this country has been cut in half, from 20,000 cases per year to approximately 10,000. It would be hard to find a more dramatic example of the benefits of improved maternal and infant care (Richmond, 1978).

Despite the better care of high-risk babies and preventive measures given in the prenatal periods, we still see infants with cerebral palsy. Further studies will have to be undertaken to determine whether there actually is a decrease or increase in certain countries.

Should Expectant Mothers Be Made Aware of the Chance of Cerebral Palsy Happening to Their Child?

It is not only the subject of cerebral palsy that should be discussed with expectant parents, but the possibility of many different problems.

A physician, nurse, physical therapist, or any other professional person involved in prenatal care may want to discuss with parents the various problems that could arise in pregnancy. Perhaps the parents may raise the question because they are more aware of potential problems that may occur during the pregnancy or the delivery.

If there is a concern about any hereditary factors, various tests may be in order to study the genetic background of the parents. Such tests would not indicate whether the child would be born with cerebral palsy but could alert the family to other conditions.

Early examinations by the obstetrician may indicate the mother has a small pelvic opening through which the fetus must pass during delivery. The possibility of a Caesarean operation may be discussed with the parents-to-be. Such discussions are not meant to put fear into the hearts of the couple but rather to make them aware that there are precautions to take and means to avoid having a high-risk infant.

No parent thinks of having a child with cerebral palsy. Knowledge of what causes cerebral palsy, mental retardation, and other developmental disabilities, however, can only enlighten the parents and cause them to be cautious during the pregnancy period. It all comes back to good prenatal care!

Can Cerebral Palsy Occur Long After Birth?

The medical literature refers to cerebral palsy as occurring in the prenatal, natal, and postnatal stages.

It is possible to have all the characteristics of the condition of cerebral palsy a long time after birth due to a particular injury, accident, or disease. When this occurs, the condition may be referred to as *acquired cerebral palsy,* rather than *congenital,* the type seen from birth.

Among the typical injuries that could cause cerebral palsy to children and adults are severe trauma due to an accident, a fall, or being struck on the head. The person who suffers from loss of oxygen due to smoke inhalation or almost drowning may show damage similar to cerebral palsy. Neoplasms or tumors can also be the cause of what would be recognized as a cerebral palsy-type condition.

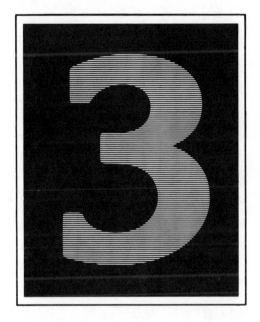

GROWTH AND
DEVELOPMENT

HANDLING THE NEW BABY

Are There Specific Techniques for Handling a Baby with Cerebral Palsy?

Despite the preparation new parents may have for caring for their baby, it is most likely that there will be special concerns in handling the infant with cerebral palsy.

If the infant was considered in the high-risk category and it becomes apparent that there is a problem, professional help should be sought in managing the child. Public health nurses, physical and occupational therapists, and those professionals involved in an early intervention program all have a contribution to make to the new parents. Anyone who has a child without a disability is aware of all that is involved in caring for a baby. The child with cerebral palsy may present all the typical baby problems plus those superimposed on the situation because of the brain damage. The infant may not be able to suck properly, making breast feeding or bottle time a difficult situation. Some infants may have a tongue thrust, a drooling problem, or be subject to severe spasticity. It will take extra patience on the part of the parents to meet these difficulties.

There are specific techniques for lifting, carrying, and bathing the child with cerebral palsy. Positioning while feeding the infant will allow for adequate control. It is important for parents to make the correct choice of a baby carriage, stroller, or chair.

To assist parents, there is an excellent publication that has received world-wide acceptance. It has been published in at least 10 languages and seems to be the most appropriate reference for parents. Check with your local library or treatment center, or purchase the publication:

Handling the Young Cerebral Palsied Child at Home by Nancie R. Finnie. E. P. Dutton, Publishers, New York (1975).

What Will My Child's Limitations Be?

This will depend upon the overall mental and physical condition of the child. Many children with cerebral palsy become self-sufficient adults, but there still are those who need varying degrees of care throughout their lives. Because of the wide range of disability involved in cerebral palsy, there is no formula to determine what limitations will be present as the child grows.

I received the following letter from a 27-year-old woman with cerebral palsy. Her letter clearly demonstrates how long it may take to determine what limitations are present.

Do you remember when we were at P.S. 135? You always said that one day I would walk. Well, you were right. It took me 21 years to realize my ability to walk, and after I realized it, there was no one to work with me. So at the age of 21, I started crawling on my hands and knees. About ten months later, I was walking with underarm crutches, until one day I went to a friend's house, and my friend had Canadian crutches. I did much better with them, so I now am able to walk some distance without anybody around me. At the age of 21, I also started to dress and undress myself, along with feeding myself. Now I am able to do almost everything on my own and with little supervision. Sometimes, I regret waiting so long before improving myself, but I guess that's the way it was meant to be. I am very happy when I take care of myself. There is a big difference in all my life now.

What Is the "Apgar Score"?

Many delivery rooms in hospitals use the Apgar Scoring System (Table 1) to rate the baby's physical condition. The infant is rated 1 minute after birth on a scale of 0 to 2 for each of five different areas. They include heart rate, respiration, reflex response, color, and muscle tone. A total score of nine or ten would indicate that the child is in fine condition. A score of four or less requires immediate intervention and often lifesaving steps. The scoring procedure is repeated 5 minutes after birth.

Table 1. Apgar Scoring Chart

Sign	0	1	2
Heart rate	Absent	Slow (below 100)	Over 100
Respiratory effort	Absent	Weak cry, hypo-ventilation	Good strong cry
Muscle tone	Limp	Some flexion of extremities	Well flexed
Reflex response (tangential foot slap)	No response	Some motion	Cry and with-drawal of foot
Color	Blue, pale	Body, pink; ex-tremities, blue	Completely pink

It is important to recognize that a low score immediately after birth may be the result of a temporary depression. There should be more concern for a marked drop in a higher score after 5 or 10 minutes. Such a drop could be associated with some permanent changes.

THE PRIMITIVE REFLEXES

What Are "Primitive Reflexes"?

Primitive reflexes are those that are developed during the growing period of the fetus while being carried by the mother. They are reflexes that are present at birth, which, in a normal child, come automatically.

A child with cerebral palsy has brain damage which either prevents the reflex from being seen or slows the appearance of the reflex. An example of a primitive reflex is sucking. A normal infant immediately after birth should be able to accept the mother's nipple and suck quite actively. If there is brain damage, there could be a negative reaction and the sucking would be limited or absent.

Another example is the Moro Reflex in which the normal infant reacts to a loud stimulus or to positioning that allows the head to fall back. The normal response would involve movement of the arms and bending of the elbows. If this does not occur or occurs in an excessive degree, the examiner may consider the possibility that there has been some damage to the nervous system.

As the infant develops, the primitive reflexes disappear and other postural reflexes come into play. There are anticipated time periods for primitive reflexes to give way to other growth and postural reflexes as described in Table 2.

In reading the chart, the + sign indicates that the reflex is positive or present. The 0 indicates the reflex is absent. The combination of the + and − signs means that the reflex is in a transitional stage or a change-over period.

Table 2. Basic reflexes from birth to 36 months of age

Reflex	Months										
	1	2	3	4	6	9	12	15	18	24	36
Palmar grasp	+	+	±	±	0[a]	0	0	0	0	0	0
Asymmetrical tonic neck	+	+	±	±	0	0	0	0	0	0	0
Moro	+	+	±	±	0	0	0	0	0	0	0
Reciprocal kicking	±	+	+	±	±	±	0	0	0	0	0
Rooting and sucking	+	+	+	+	+	±	0[b]	0	0	0	0
Neck righting (two-step)	0	0	0	±	±	+	+	+	+	+	+
Parachute (protective extension of arms)	0	0	0	0	±	+	+	+	+	+	+
Landau (head up—back arched a bit in ventral suspension)	0	0	0	0	0	±	+	±	±	±	0

[a]Reflex grasp may still be present in sleep.
[b]Rooting and sucking may still be present when hungry or asleep.

The neck righting, parachute, and Landau reflexes would be considered in the postural category and are not seen in early infancy.

Any problems with the primitive or postural reflexes should be observed by your pediatrician because they could indicate a need for further neurological examination.

What Is the "Fencing Position"?

The fencing position actually describes a reflex that is present at birth known as the asymmetrical tonic neck reflex (ATNR). It usually is seen from infancy through about 6 months of age. If it continues in any excessive degree after 5 months, it can be used as an index of suspicion that the child may have some type of neurological problem.

For this position, the infant should be on his or her back. By turning the head approximately 45 degrees to one side, the arm on that side will extend or straighten out as will the leg on the same side.

On the opposite side, the arm will flex or bend, as will the leg. If this persists, as the child reaches the age when sitting starts, it could interfere with getting into a sitting position or eventual standing. Children who are developing normally, though slowly, however, do overcome the automatic response and do progress to sitting, standing, or walking.

Why Do Some Children Sit Earlier Than Others?

Child development studies demonstrate that a child must have enough strength in the neck and back to overcome the force of gravity and sit alone. In normal growth, sitting alone for long periods of time comes at approximately 40 weeks. Some children may mature a bit earlier and others later. The lack of sitting for very short periods with some support at 6 months could be cause for suspicion of a problem. The child with cerebral palsy may have a developmental delay and be slow to mature. Here again, some children with cerebral palsy will accomplish certain activities at different stages and times. Because no two children are exactly alike, you can expect some will assume a sitting position without support before others.

Is Sitting Learned in a Child with Cerebral Palsy or Does It Come When the Brain Says So?

Sitting alone and unsupported occurs by 9 or 10 months in a normal child. It is an expected stage of development.

With the child with cerebral palsy, the various developmental stages do not occur at the anticipated time. The child's maturation and developmental schedule is disturbed. Preparation for sitting may occur through the use of basic postural patterns used by physical and occupational therapists in neurodevelopmental techniques (NDT).

By Looking At an Infant with Cerebral Palsy, Can You Tell How Severe the Disability Will Be in the Future?

It is extremely difficult to picture what the infant with cerebral palsy will look like 5 years later. The pediatrician, in particular, is often asked this question by parents who want some assurance that their child will continue to be only mildly impaired if, at infancy, the signs of cerebral palsy are minimal. Such may not be the case because development related to sitting and walking may change the appearance of the child. Dr. Kenneth S. Holt (1979), Professor of Developmental Pediatrics at the University of London, stated, "In current medical practice and training, the skill of diagnosis receives great attention and the art of prognosis very little."

Dr. Holt suggests that there have been situations in which the pediatrician may have told the parents to expect little from the child only to be quite surprised when the child returned for examination several years later. He suggests that the parents give the child as good a training program as possible for several years; then upon re-examination, a better picture of the child's future can be obtained. Parents who may have observed the lack of development in their child over such a period are more likely to accept a "cautious outlook" if that is what is called for.

Are Most Children with Cerebral Palsy the First Born in the Family?

Several studies have been done to determine the frequency of cerebral palsy in firstborn children. In one major study reported by Cruickshank (1976) conducted in New Jersey, 24.5% of the children with cerebral palsy were the first in order of birth and the result of the first pregnancy. The second pregnancy and second in order of birth accounted for 29.8% of the group in that study.

Cerebral palsy may be related to any or all pregnancies. There is no apparent evidence at present to demonstrate that there is a strong tendency for children with cerebral palsy to be the first born.

How Is the Denver Developmental Screening Test Used in Cerebral Palsy?

The Denver Developmental Screening Test (DDST) provides a simple, clinically useful tool for the early detection of children who may be significantly developmentally delayed. According to Haynes (1979), the test can be given in 10 to 20 minutes to children from the ages of 1 month to 6 years.

The test is designed to assess development in four major areas: gross motor, language, fine motor-adaptive, and personal-social.

The application of the DDST can be very significant in working with children with cerebral palsy or those suspected of having a problem.

If you have any concerns about the test, this should be discussed with professional personnel at your treatment facility.

Should the Denver Pre-Screening Developmental Questionnaire Be Used Before the DDST?

It has been reported that using the Denver Pre-Screening Developmental Questionnaire (PDQ) has reduced the need to administer the full Denver test by 69% (Haynes, 1979).

The questionnaire was developed as a tool that could be given to parents to get information about the child. Parents are asked to respond to 10 developmental questions related to the child's abilities. It can be completed in a very short time (about 5 minutes).

The PDQ is economical and one learns to administer it very quickly. Parents seem to like the PDQ because it helps them to be more aware of the developmental progress of their children (Haynes, 1979).

What Is the Brazelton Assessment Scale?

The Brazelton Neonatal Behavioral Assessment Scale may be used to detect abnormalities while the infant is still in the hospital. The scale is of value not only in promoting early detection of abnormality but also in developing insight about each baby's individual repertoire of behaviors (Haynes, 1979).

The scale explores the infant's responses on 27 different dimensions. It can be administered once the infant reaches initial stability and can be repeated on succeeding days. Some of the areas in which responses are recorded include reaction to light, sounds, and visual stimulation, muscle tone and motor maturity, cuddling, and excitement.

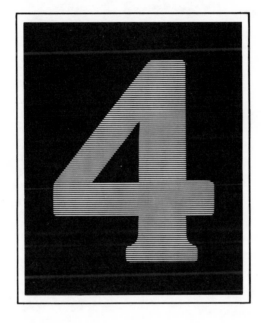

MEDICAL AND
SURGICAL PROBLEMS

Does the Condition of Cerebral Palsy Render a Person More Susceptible to Common Colds or Flu, or to Childhood Diseases?

"When my cerebral palsied child came down with chicken-pox, I realized how normal she was," a parent told this author. Children with cerebral palsy are subject to all of the typical childhood diseases as would be any child. The seriousness of a cold or the flu may be dependent, however, upon the severity of the child's handicap. Those with respiratory problems will find it more difficult to overcome the common cold or the flu. The severely handicapped child may also be more susceptible to what many normal people take for granted, only because the child does not have the general strength to fight such illnesses. Even a common cold may be difficult for the severely involved child and medical attention may be necessary. In the early 1950s, pneumonia was a major problem for children with cerebral palsy. Rothman (1978) suggests that a treatment plan for improving motor control in children with cerebral palsy should also include the teaching of breathing exercises to help increase breathing capacity and decrease the likelihood of lung infections.

As Children with Cerebral Palsy Grow Older, Do They Develop More Problems?

Although it is accepted that cerebral palsy is a nonprogressive condition, it is very possible other problems may develop as the child grows older.

Such problems may not actually be related to the condition of cerebral palsy but may rather be superimposed upon the individual. The normal effect of growth on one's posture, balance, and ambulation must be considered. Positioning, especially for the nonambulatory child, should receive attention in order to prevent spinal deformities, such as scoliosis.

Emotional problems often develop when the teenager with cerebral palsy recognizes a lack of social acceptance from members of the so-called normal society. The lack of ability to cope with major adolescent changes may be very disturbing to the teenager.

Frustrations resulting from the inability to obtain a higher education or gainful and meaningful employment can become a major problem.

In addition, adults with cerebral palsy will be subject to the same physical aging process as everyone else.

SURGICAL PROCEDURES

What Is the Value in Doing a Heel Cord Lengthening in a Young Child with Cerebral Palsy?

When a young child with cerebral palsy continuously walks on the toes, it may be an indication that this child has a tight heel cord. This would be recognized by your physician. Surgical correction in the form of a tendon lengthening is often done after more conservative methods do not relieve the problem. Such methods may include night splints, bracing, stretching, and physical therapy. A recurrence of the problem is often seen if the surgery is done at an early age.

In a major study (Lee and Bleck, 1980) in which 67 children with cerebral palsy had been operated on, data showed that patients who had surgery at an early age were most prone to recurrence of the problem. In Lee and Bleck's report, the doctors state, "Because the more severely involved children develop contractures earlier, they had surgery earlier; therefore, with the potential for more years of growth, recurrence may be more likely." Their data did not imply that surgery should be delayed until the child is older.

The heel-cord lengthening procedure is often done to improve the child's walking ability, to help in giving better balance, and to prevent further deformity from taking place.

What Should Be Done
After A Heel Cord Lengthening?

Postoperative care for the child who undergoes the surgical procedure known as a heel cord lengthening has traditionally included bracing, night splinting, and heel cord stretching. Usually, the parents are shown how to do the heel cord stretching and instructed to follow a planned time for the activity. For the very young child, the parent will find it most opportune to do the stretching activities during bath time.

Recently, two orthopedists (Lee and Bleck, 1980) suggested a change in the approach to the surgical procedure. They believe that it is unnecessary to subject the patient and family to hours of heel cord stretching, using special shoes, or night splints as the child grows. They suggest that the child be free of medical care and given the opportunity to have mobility in play. Six weeks after surgery, after the plaster cast is removed, Drs. Lee and Bleck recommend that ordinary soft shoes or tennis shoes be used and supervised physical therapy with the emphasis on gait and balance training be integrated with the activities of daily living.

Not all orthopedic surgeons will agree with this approach and because there may be differences of opinion related to the heel cord lengthening procedure, this should be discussed with your chosen physician before the surgery takes place.

What Is an Adductor Tenotomy?

A tenotomy is the surgical section (or cutting) of a tendon. When referring to the adductors, this implies the surgical procedure will be done on the muscle or muscle group that brings the legs together.

Should it be determined by the physician that the adductors are causing deformities or are interfering with ambulation, a surgical procedure may be suggested. The selection of the procedure and a well-planned follow up with physical therapy should be discussed thoroughly with the parents.

What Is the "Brain Pacemaker"?

In 1972, Dr. Irving Cooper's surgical implantation of electrodes on the cerebellum was a major advance in treating certain cerebral palsy conditions. The electrodes are stimulated by a radio transmitter which is carried outside of the body by way of a radio-frequency receiver implanted in the person's chest. Although the term *brain pacemaker* has been adopted by the press, it actually does not truly describe the instrument. According to United Cerebral Palsy's Foundation Medical Director, Dr. Leon Sternfeld, the correct term is *chronic cerebellar stimulation,* more commonly referred to as a *CCS.*

How Popular Is Use of CCS?

Over a period of 6 years from 1972 through 1978, some 700 persons have undergone the procedure. Extensive research is still being conducted to determine the long-range effect of the system. Although the procedure has demonstrated improvement in some areas, a conservative approach has been taken on recommending general application to many persons until further studies are completed. It still is experimental!

How Costly Is the CCS Procedure?

It takes a specialist (neurosurgeon) and a medical team to carry out the implant procedure. Third-party funding through medical plans and insurance has not generally been available for payment. Costs run between an estimated $8,000 to $16,000 and more.

Can Brain Damage Be Repaired?

With the knowledge and techniques presently used in the treatment of cerebral palsy, there is no way of repairing damage that has occurred to the brain.

SEIZURES AND DRUG CONTROL

Do All Persons with Cerebral Palsy Necessarily Have Seizures?

No. Several major studies involving some 3,000 persons with cerebral palsy demonstrate that the possibility of the child having epilepsy varies considerably. In the three studies the range was from 14% to 40%.

One researcher found convulsions to be three times as great in spastic children as in children with athetosis. Another study indicated that 50% of all children who were diagnosed as being in the spastic classification had seizures, compared to 15% with athetosis (Cruikshank, 1976; p. 23).

Because epilepsy can result from brain injury before, during, or after birth, the possibility of a child with cerebral palsy having seizures should not be overlooked.

The Epilepsy Foundation of America (1981a) estimates that four million Americans have some form of epilepsy.

What Is an "Aura"?

The person with epilepsy may experience a warning of some type just before the onset of the seizure. This warning may come in various forms, such as a buzzing in the ear, an uneasiness, or a peculiar feeling in the stomach. The person may recognize a particular odor or see a certain color.

The aura is an indication of the coming seizure. Appropriate steps should immediately be taken to protect the individual as the seizure develops.

How Would One Notice a Mild Seizure?

There are many different types of epileptic seizures. Noticing a very mild seizure may be difficult if you are not aware of certain characteristics.

The "petit mal," generally associated with young children, is characterized by short blinking or staring for just a few seconds. These little seizures may occur seldom to often throughout the day. The person is usually not aware of the seizures.

The parents may notice a blank expression or see that the child appears to pay no attention to what is going on in the surroundings. If this type of seizure is suspected, parents should keep a close record and by all means look to a physician for treatment of the child.

Petit mal seizures may disappear at puberty, but they can also continue through adulthood with less severity.

It has been reported that the petit mal or mildest of seizures almost never occurs in children with cerebral palsy (Downey and Low, 1974).

Will the Seizures Ever Stop?

Seizures can be controlled in most cases when the child with cerebral palsy is under the medical supervision of a physician and certain medications (anticonvulsants) are prescribed.

Some young children may develop an occasional seizure that appears to have no cause. These seizures do not persist over a long period of time.

It appears that most seizures in children with cerebral palsy start at between 2 and 6 years of age. The most common type of seizure is the "grand mal" which is subject to control through medication.

What Are Infantile Myoclonic Spasms?

Infantile myoclonic spasms are a form of epilepsy seen in young children usually in the first 3 years of life. Such seizures may first be noticed at 4 to 6 months of age. The seizures last only a few seconds but may be seen throughout the day. They often are replaced by more serious types of seizures as the child grows older, and they may lead to serious retardation.

The spasms are recognized by the sudden flexion or bending of the arms and trunk with stiffening of the legs. The hands tend to meet the bowed head similar to what one would see in a far-eastern nation's method of greeting another person. Perhaps for this reason, the seizures are often referred to as *salaam seizures.*

After the attack, the child usually will cry and the eyes may have a fixed stare. During the attack, the child may lose color, breathe rapidly, and tend to sweat. Such attacks seem to appear more often when the child is tired and drowsy or when waking up.

What Are the Long-Term Effects of the Continued Use of Dilantin? . . . of Tegretol?

Dilantin is an anticonvulsant agent often prescribed for those with cerebral palsy to aid in the control of seizures. It has been demonstrated that continued use leads to such side effects as slurred speech, confusion, involuntary eyeball movements, dizziness, and nervousness.

Most common to children and adults with cerebral palsy who have been on Dilantin for long periods is a condition in which the gums grow over the teeth. This is known as *hyperplasia* (see page 69 on hyperplasia).

Tegretol, another anticonvulsant drug, often causes nausea, dizziness, drowsiness, and vomiting when first given as a treatment for control of seizures. Close supervision by a physician is recommended for those using this medication. The manufacturer also suggests blood counts, liver function tests, urinalysis, and eye examinations be carried out at regular intervals.

What Effect Does Phenobarbital Have on Children?

"Phenobarb" is a long-acting barbiturate used as a daytime sedative and is often prescribed for the management of epilepsy. Continued use may produce inconsistent excitement and hyperactivity in children.

Phenobarbital is another drug that requires close medical supervision. Such supervision takes on added importance when the child or adult with cerebral palsy is undergoing stress due to major changes in the environment such as starting in a new school, going for a vacation at a camp, or seeking employment.

If My Child with Cerebral Palsy Is Subject to Seizures, Should Surgery Be Considered to Eliminate Them?

There are several conditions that should be met before considering surgery for any child with cerebral palsy and epilepsy.

In an article in the *National Spokesman,* issued by the Epilepsy Foundation of America (1981), the following information was given when surgery is an option.

> Although many criteria are involved in a physician's recommendation for or against surgery as a treatment for epilepsy, the following are some of the conditions that must be met:
>
> . . . It must be possible to identify seizure activity as originating in a single, relatively small, area of the brain.
> . . . This area must be so located that its removal would not endanger other vital brain functions.
> . . . Treatment with standard anticonvulsants has proved ineffective.
>
> A small number of specialized centers currently offer this type of surgery in the United States. (p. 5)

Can Persons with Cerebral Palsy Obtain Special Discounts on Drugs?

If parents or the adult with cerebral palsy is employed in a situation in which there is a drug plan, there would be discounts on prescriptions ordered by a physician.

If a person with cerebral palsy is in need of drugs for control of seizures, it would be worthwhile to be a member of the Epilepsy Foundation of America. For more information, write to:

> Epilepsy Foundation of America
> 4351 Garden City Drive
> Landover, MD 20785

CLASSIFICATIONS

How Do You Recognize Hemiplegia?

Hemiplegia, as a term, describes the involvement of both extremities on the same side, such as the left arm and left leg. Children with spastic paralysis of a mild to moderate degree often are found to be hemiplegic.

This term may also be associated with an individual who suffers from a stroke or cardiovascular accident (CVA).

What Do the Terms *Quadriplegia,* *Tetraplegia,* and *Diplegia* Mean?

These terms are used when all four extremities (the arms and the legs) are involved with a handicapping condition such as cerebral palsy.

You often hear the term *quadriplegia* when reference is made to a person who has suffered a severe injury to the vertebrae of the neck, damaging the spinal cord and involving both arms and legs. The child with cerebral palsy whose brain damage affects the motor control of all four extremities may also be classified as quadriplegic.

Tetraplegia also refers to involvement in all four extremities.

The term *diplegia* is sometimes used to indicate the lower extremities are more severely involved than the upper extremities.

Are Paraplegics Always Confined to a Wheelchair?

The term "paraplegic" has gained much attention since films have been made of veterans returning from various wars with injuries resulting in their using wheelchairs. The injuries are not the same as seen in cerebral palsy, but the terminology applies.

Paraplegia is a term used when the lower extremities are affected in any manner. You often will see a child or adult with cerebral palsy, who may be classified as having paraplegia, using some form of crutches or a walker for ambulation. It will depend upon the severity of the condition of cerebral palsy. The more severely involved person with spastic paraplegia may be confined to a wheelchair.

According to Dr. and Mrs. Bobath (1975) true paraplegias are very rare in cerebral palsy. Very few children show no involvement "above the waist" as seen in spinal injuries. The more common paralysis associated with cerebral palsy is diplegia, with mild involvement of arms and hands, sometimes only of one arm.

Is There Something Known As a "CP Squint"?

A major medical dictionary defines "squint" as being synonymous with strabismus, a defect in which the child is unable to direct both eyes at the same time toward a point.

Statistics from several studies of children with cerebral palsy show that squint was found in a wide range of children, from 17% to 60%. The fact that squint is so prominent emphasizes the importance of opthalmological evaluations as part of the total assessment of the child's condition. Such evaluations should be done as early as possible to prevent loss of vision in the deviant or problem eye and further visual problems.

SCOLIOSIS

What Is Scoliosis?

The term *scoliosis* is often used to generally describe any curvature of the spine. It is not a disease or disorder but a deformity that can be brought about for many reasons and at different ages.

In classifying the condition, parents should be familiar with the term *idiopathic*. This refers to any condition brought on without a clear recognizable cause. Idiopathic scoliosis may occur from birth to 3 years of age and is considered "infantile." This type appears to be more common in boys.

The juvenile type of scoliosis appears from 4 years of age to 9 years. Girls seem more prone to this type than boys. The adolescent condition appears from 10 years to the end of the growth period. It is more common in girls than in boys.

The idiopathic type of structural scoliosis comprises about 85% of the disorder and may develop in otherwise healthy, normal children and adolescents.

Progression of the condition is the major concern. Treatment varies but may include a combination of correction of the curvature and surgical stabilization. More moderate cases may only require some type of corrective plaster casting and bracing.

Most important in the treatment of scoliosis is early recognition, diagnosis, and effective orthopedic treatment.

Do Many Children with Cerebral Palsy Have Scoliosis?

Several of the major texts on cerebral palsy written in the 1960s have little or no reference to the possibilities of a child with cerebral palsy developing scoliosis.

More recently, Rinsky and Kleinman (1981) described the incidence of scoliosis in patients with cerebral palsy. Their work indicates an incidence of 5% to 7%, depending on how severe a curve one uses for the cut-off point when making a diagnosis. According to their findings, the incidence rises to 39% for severe institutionalized quadriplegic patients. They also suggest this figure may apply to the very severely handicapped person with cerebral palsy who may be found in various community programs.

How Can Scoliosis Be Prevented?

As indicated in the previous question, most cases of scoliosis occur without any specific cause. One of the major problems seen in children and adults with cerebral palsy is poor posture. This may lead to an actual structural deformity.

In particular, the child or adult with cerebral palsy confined to a wheelchair for most of the day, must be positioned so that movement can be undertaken without placing undue strain and constant pressure on the spine. The child who constantly leans to one side of the wheelchair, with little support for maintaining an upright position, is a likely candidate for scoliosis. The spinal curve that develops will lead to numerous problems, including interference with the breathing process. Preventive care is available by customizing the wheelchair and being sure appropriate inserts keep the child comfortable. Opportunities to change position and leave the wheelchair should be offered as often as possible.

As the child with cerebral palsy grows, watch for any structural changes in the spinal column. This will also be a concern to professional personnel working with the child.

Prevention of severe scoliosis due to poor posture and positioning is a possibility. Medical examinations on a periodic basis are also important.

What Are the Goals of Surgery in Scoliosis?

The goals of surgical treatment in spinal deformities are always primarily functional. These include (according to Rinsky and Kleinman, 1981) the following:

1. The ability to sit or be seated with hands free
2. Freedom from back pain
3. The ability to breathe more easily

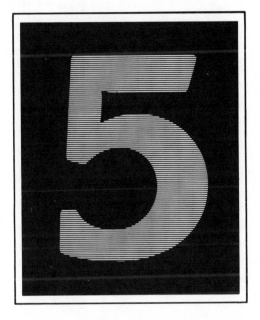

PROFESSIONAL
SERVICES

Do Adults with Cerebral Palsy Need Regular Medical Checkups?

Regular medical checkups are absolutely necessary for adults (as well as children) with cerebral palsy. The checkups are most important if the person is taking any kind of medication. In addition, because many of the adults with cerebral palsy seem to be less active than nondisabled people, they could be subject to more medical problems.

For those adults with cerebral palsy known to a treatment service organization that offers medical and therapeutic programs, checkups should be relatively easy to obtain.

If no extensive services are available to the adult with cerebral palsy in the immediate neighborhood, it is most worthwhile to make one's presence known to a local physician just in case an emergency need ever presents itself.

Are There Any Doctors Who Specialize in the Treatment of Cerebral Palsy?

In 1947, a group of physicians concerned with developing interest in cerebral palsy, formed the American Academy for Cerebral Palsy. The organization grew and today membership in the Academy consists of hundreds of professionals who have a significant interest in cerebral palsy and other developmental disorders.

Further information on such specialists may be obtained by writing the Academy:

American Academy for Cerebral Palsy
and Developmental Medicine
P.O. Box 11083
Richmond, VA 23230

In addition, information on special services for persons with cerebral palsy may be obtained through:

The Easter Seal Society
2020 West Ogden Ave.
Chicago, IL 60612

or

United Cerebral Palsy Associations, Inc.
66 East 34 St.
New York, NY 10016

How Soon Should Treatment Be Started?

Even before a definite diagnosis of cerebral palsy is made, treatment should be started to reach the child at his or her particular developmental level. This may be in the form of an "early intervention" program in which the child receives all types of stimulation and the parents are involved in the total program.

Early treatment is important because of the great adaptability and plasticity of the infantile brain (Bobath, 1967). It is well known that the first 18 months of a normal child's life involves tremendous and rapid growth and development. For children with cerebral palsy it is also a time for adjustment to cerebral damage.

A 7-year study in the North Carolina Cerebral Palsy Hospital (1979), suggests that the sooner the treatment program is begun, the better. With the services that are available today in so many communities, there is little reason to wait until the child is 2 or 3 years of age before initiating some well-programmed activities.

If the child is unable to participate in a formalized program, parents should be instructed on how best to help the child in a home program. Both the mother and the father should be aware of instruction available from qualified personnel. The parents should be able to carry out a routine program in the home. Because the child with cerebral palsy may not be able to be involved in the normal activities any other child would encounter, the parents will have to set up a stimulating environment to meet the child's needs. (see page 72).

Although early treatment has received support from many sources, there is no actual proof that such an approach is the right way to handle all children with cerebral palsy. Because such intervention apparently cannot hurt the child, however, a program would be worthwhile in support of the parent's desire to help their child.

Does Treatment Cure Cerebral Palsy?

Cure, according to Webster's Dictionary has been defined as "the restoration to health or a sound condition." At present, there is no known cure for cerebral palsy.

Treatment can bring about changes and prevent the condition from interfering with the activities of normal living. Treatment will depend on what functional impairments are noted.

The various approaches to the care, management, and treatment of children with cerebral palsy offer training that may improve the control of different aspects of the condition.

As parents, do not look for any miracle cure to totally eliminate cerebral palsy. Early intervention and a treatment program based on assessment and evaluation are the important factors in helping a child to take part in as many fulfilling and enjoyable experiences as possible in spite of cerebral palsy.

How Do You Know If the Child Needs Different Types of Care and Programming?

The typical approach to determining what children with cerebral palsy need is through a thorough developmental assessment and evaluation. This may be combined with early intervention even before a definite diagnosis of cerebral palsy is made.

In the evaluation process, the child will be observed by a team of special professional personnel that may include (but not be limited to) the pediatrician, nurse, psychologist, teacher, speech pathologist, physical therapist, occupational therapist, and social worker. Members of the team, working closely with the parents, carefully evaluate all aspects of sensory and motor development.

In an early intervention program, when deficits or delays in growth and development of the child are found, the team may make specific recommendations for further professional input and programming.

Out of this total approach will come the most appropriate program for the child. The program is subject to review periodically as the child develops, matures, and progresses and as new environmental opportunities become available.

What Is the Purpose of Braces?

When ordered for a child with cerebral palsy, braces have several different purposes, primarily:

1. To prevent deformity
2. To give support
3. To control movement

Braces act primarily on the joint that is crossed. For example, a short-leg brace that inserts into the heel of the shoe will act only on the ankle, as it does not go over the knee.

A full-length brace may control the foot, knee, and hip and have an extension to support the back. Braces require a great deal of care, exact measurement for comfort, and they are quite expensive.

During the 1940s and 1950s, braces were most popular in the treatment and management of children with cerebral palsy.

DENTAL

What Happens When My Child Gets Cavities?

Even with good dental hygiene, it is likely that your child will go through the normal stages of getting cavities. Be prepared by checking with your family dentist to find out if children with disabilities can be handled in the dental office.

A child with mild cerebral palsy should be able to be serviced by any dentist. Children with cerebral palsy should have the benefit of dentistry provided under normal conditions, both in private offices and special clinics (Rosenstein, 1978).

It has been recognized by leading dental authorities that, with repeated visits to the dental office and concern demonstrated by dental personnel, most of the children and adults with cerebral palsy will be able to understand the need for cooperation.

Various dental instruments have also been adapted for use when working with disabled children and adults, thus making most standard dental procedures possible.

Do Many Dentists Treat Handicapped Patients?

A special report on *Dental Care for Handicapped Americans* (Robert Woods Foundation, 1979) estimates that between 10% and 25% of the nation's 115,000 practicing dentists indicate a willingness to treat certain kinds of handicapped patients. Unfortunately, despite the willingness, many dentists are unable to serve those persons with cerebral palsy because of the patient's severe disability or for such reasons as related architectural barriers which prevent access to dental facilities.

The report has hope for the future. It states, "the number of dentists with the skills and the commitment to treat handicapped persons is slowly on the increase."

If you need dental services for your handicapped child, check with your local dental society, nearest hospital facility, or the Cerebral Palsy Association.

Do All Children and Adults with Cerebral Palsy in Need of Dental Services Require General Anesthesia?

Studies by Green and Mendelsohn (1960) indicated the need for premedication of children and adults with cerebral palsy was greatly below expectations. Any person with cerebral palsy in need of extensive dental care may be subject to extreme fear and anxiety. Time must be taken by dental personnel and the parents of the individual with cerebral palsy to alleviate or reduce such problems. The extra time required to handle some of the patients with cerebral palsy may not always be available at your local practitioner's office.

It is important to look into what services are available through your treatment facility or local cerebral palsy center.

Should your child's disability be so severe as to need general anesthesia for dental work, this usually is done with the cooperation of a well-equipped medical facility.

Do Children and Adults with Cerebral Palsy Require More Dental Services Than Other People?

Services related to dentistry for persons with cerebral palsy are similar to those needed by anyone else. They all require the usual x-rays, diagnosis, fillings, extractions, dental hygiene, and some appliances. Older children with cerebral palsy may require orthodontic treatment and replacements. Periodontal treatments and certain appliances are frequently required for adults with cerebral palsy.

Prevention is an important issue with disabled persons. Often neglect and the inability to obtain dental services lead to problems.

In general, it is found that children with cerebral palsy are susceptible to the same oral and dental diseases and disorders as are other children, but there is a greater degree of susceptibility to disorders of the supporting structures and occlusion (relation of the teeth when the jaws are closed) than in normal children (Rosenstein, 1978).

Are There Special Facilities Offering Dental Services to Persons with Cerebral Palsy?

Some major hospitals and medical centers maintain specialty clinics for the physically and mentally handicapped.

Although there has been increasing attention given to the dental problems of children and adults with cerebral palsy, there are areas in which services may be limited. It would be best to check with your local dental society to determine what facilities are available or which dentists may have a speciality in working with the handicapped.

The National Foundation of Dentistry for the Handicapped, a Denver based organization, operates 78 participating facilities in Colorado. By the fall of 1979, the foundation was operating in eight states. The ultimate goal of the group is to be active in all 50 states. For further information write:

> The National Foundation of Dentistry
> for the Handicapped
> 1726 Champa, Suite 442
> Denver, CO 80202

In the New York City area, the Dental Guidance Council for Cerebral Palsy has been a forerunner in establishing services for the handicapped. Currently, national promotion is underway. For information write:

> United Cerebral Palsy Associations, Inc.
> 66 East 34 Street
> New York, NY 10036

What Is Hyperplasia?

Hyperplasia refers to the excessive growth of normal cells in the tissue arrangements of an organ. More specifically, in people with cerebral palsy, hyperplasia refers to the condition in which the gums tend to grow over the teeth. This is related to the continued use of the anticonvulsant drug, Dilantin. Dental researchers attribute the problem to the dose and serum levels of the drug.

For a free booklet, *Phenytoin (Dilantin) and Dental Care,* write to:

> Epilepsy Foundation of America
> 4351 Garden City Drive
> Landover, MD 20785

What Can Be Done for the Child with Hyperplasia?

Good dental care and oral hygiene are a must for the child with hyperplasia. Frequent dental checks should be part of the total management program for the child.

It is imperative that the child or adult with cerebral palsy using the drug Dilantin, a prime cause of hyperplasia, should be under the supervision of a physician.

Can Adults with Cerebral Palsy Use Dentures?

Generally, adults with cerebral palsy who are severely physically involved are not ideal subjects for dentures. Emphasis should be placed on good dental hygiene to prevent the need for dentures. The dentist trained to care for the handicapped, however, may be able to successfully meet the needs of some adults by using innovative approaches to the fitting and placement of dentures.

PODIATRIC

What Is an Orthosis?

In the October 1981 issue of *The Exceptional Parent,* Fletcher and Fredrick define an orthosis as "a device that replaces a function (such as a structural support needed for walking) or provides resistance against deformity that often results from spasticity, paralysis or atrophy."

Another definition may be found in Dorland's Medical Dictionary, "Orthosis is an orthopedic appliance or apparatus used to support, align, prevent or correct deformities or to improve the function of movable parts of the body." Examples include braces and special shoes.

What Custom Foot Orthoses Are Available?

If required, many different types of custom foot orthoses are available today based on a complete static and functional examination of your child's legs and feet.

It is important that the cast be taken while the foot and leg above is being held in a position of maximal function thereby assisting the overall stability of the patient.

The design and materials, selected by your doctor, range from leather to a multitude of long-wearing, space-age thermoplastics depending on the goal of the orthosis. (P. Jordan, personal communication).

Are Orthotic Devices Usually Covered by Third Party Payments?

Third party payments usually are not received for prescription shoes, shoe modifications, or arch supports. More and more insurance companies, however, including those federally and state subsidized, and physically handicapped children's programs offer reimbursement for services rendered and for prescribed biomechanical foot orthoses.

Check with your medical insurance company for its policies and coverage.

What Is the Role of the Podiatrist in Treatment of Persons with Cerebral Palsy?

Paul Jordan, Director of Biomechanics and Rehabilitative Medicines, The Langer Group, responded to this question in a personal communication of November 17, 1981. He directed his answer to the lay person or parents of a cerebral palsied youngster.

> The "flatfoot" that you might observe in one foot and often both feet in your youngster might be a contributory factor to the overall standing/walking stability since this is the base of support for the entire body. This in turn, may aggravate the child's abnormal muscle tone.
> To find out if your child's foot posture might be aggravating his stance or walking patterns, a consultation with a podiatrist experienced in pediatric foot disorders might be advisable. A foot orthosis would be recommended if the foot has compensated for other bone or muscle "imbalances" within the lower limbs. A foot orthosis is not to be confused

with "arch supports" or "cookies" which are ineffective and often painful to wear. A foot orthosis might be employed to offer a more stable base on which to stand or walk and assist in the development of the leg alone.

How Would One Find a Podiatrist Familiar with Cerebral Palsy?

Being a relatively new medical specialty, the Pediatric Podiatrist, (podopediatrics) is rather difficult to find because they are few in number. If you contact the groups listed below, you will receive assistance in locating a podiatrist in your region familiar with pediatric foot and walking disorders.

The American Academy of Podopediatrics
c/o Ohio College of Podiatrics
10515 Carnegy Ave.
Cleveland, OH 44106

The Langer Foundation for Gait Research
21 Industry Ct.
Deer Park, NY 11729

NUTRITIONAL

What Role Does Nutrition Play in the Development of a Person with Cerebral Palsy?

Many articles have been written on the need for good nutrition for the growing child. Such concern applies to children with cerebral palsy as well. With the increased energy expenditure of children or adults with athetosis or the additional efforts required for the person with spasticity, attention must be given to the nutritional needs through life. This is also important for the child or adult with cerebral palsy who is not mobile and whose activity is severely limited.

A pediatrician should make parents aware of the role of nutrition in raising children with cerebral palsy. For proper guidance parents may also look to their treatment center where a nutritionist may be a consulting member of the staff. Overall, nutrition should be part of the total management plan established for the person with cerebral palsy.

Should the Adult with Cerebral Palsy Be Concerned About Diet and Nutrition?

Nutrition should be a concern for the adult with cerebral palsy just as with the growing child. In many situations, the adult may be confined to a wheelchair. This would result in reduced activity and a tendency to be overweight or obese. This, in turn, would make movement more difficult and reduce the adult's opportunity for independent activities. The adult with many involuntary movements, as seen in athetosis, may require more than the average amount of caloric intake. Consultation with a nutritionist or registered dietician may be just as important as regular medical checkups.

TREATMENT APPROACHES: PHYSICAL, OCCUPATIONAL, SPEECH, AND RECREATIONAL THERAPY

How Does the Therapist Predict What a Child Can or Cannot Do in Later Life?

It is very difficult (if not impossible) for any professional person to actually predict what the child with cerebral palsy will be like in years ahead. No two children are the same. Even with years of experience, the professional should be very cautious about making any statements to a parent that would suggest how the child will look or act in many years.

Some professional personnel, especially therapists, after working with the young child for many months, will recognize the lack of development in such areas as motor coordination and head control. These can be signs of additional problems that will make the child more difficult to handle in years to come.

The total picture of growth and development, together with the intellectual ability, emotional behavior, and training, will affect the child. If one sees the child is progressing on a developmental scale similar to non-cerebral palsied children, one may suggest that the child should be doing certain activities at a specific time. This can also present quite a problem to the parents if the child does not reach a certain point of development when the therapist said he or she would.

Parents will have to depend upon physicians and therapists and the educators for direction, but parents should not expect anyone to be able to give a firm prediction for the future development of the child with cerebral palsy.

Is It Important That a Child with Cerebral Palsy Spend Much Time Out of the Wheelchair?

Yes. Whenever possible, the wheelchair should be used primarily for transportation. A child confined to a wheelchair does not have an opportunity to use much of his or her body. Usually such a child is restrained to prevent falling out of the chair. Although this is done for safety, restraints also limit the child's less harmful movements.

The wheelchair may be fitted with a lap-board or tray for use as a table or a desk. This also limits movement. When opportunities are presented for the child to be out of the wheelchair, take advantage of them.

If a mat or a carpeted floor is available, the child should be placed on the mat and allowed to express himself by whatever movements are possible.

Confinement to a wheelchair can lead to deformities. Positioning should be checked by the physical therapist or the occupational therapist. Frequent checking will prevent pressure sores and be helpful in reducing the chances of scoliosis developing. Use of orthopedic aids such as crutches or walkers should be encouraged in between use of the wheelchair.

The wheelchair may be absolutely necessary for covering long distances while in the community, at school, or at a treatment center. Parents will find most of the professional personnel in the educational or treatment facility very will-ing to use special adapted equipment and not always depend on the wheelchair.

At home, parents will find many opportunities for the child to be out of the wheelchair. Placement on a soft couch, a protected corner, or an adapted chair are alternatives to the constant use of the wheelchair.

What Is NDT?

NDT is the abbreviation for the term *neurodevelopmental treatment.*

The concept formulated by Dr. and Mrs. Bobath is often referred to as the "Bobath approach". It is based on the recognition of the importance of two factors (as described in the writings of Berte Bobath, 1973):

1. The interference of normal maturation of the brain by the lesion leading to retardation or arrest of motor develop-ment
2. The presence of abnormal patterns of posture and move-ment, due to a release of abnormal postural reflex ac-tivity

The aim of neurodevelopmental treatment is to obtain changes in postural tone and patterns toward the more normal.

In many treatment centers for cerebral palsy, you will find NDT involves many disciplines and is the main ap-proach to treatment, especially of the very young child with cerebral palsy.

What Is the "Patterning" Technique?

The theory behind "patterning" is that failure to pass through the appropriate sequence of development reflects poor neurological organization. The proponents of pattern-ing, introduced by the Institutes for the Achievement of Human Potential, Philadelphia, seek to draw a response from the damaged child by introducing intense stimuli. The technique includes repeated manipulation of the head and extremities (usually involving several people), sensory stimulation, breathing exercises, restriction of fluid intake, early learning of reading, and other techniques used to establish brain hemispheric dominance. The names of the director and associate director of the Institutes, Glenn Doman and Carl Delacato, are often used in referring to the patterning program.

"Patterning" as a treatment approach has not been universally and exclusively accepted by all professional personnel in treatment centers. This approach (as well as other techniques) should be discussed with your physician and therapists.

What Are Some of the Other Approaches to the Treatment of Children with Cerebral Palsy?

The neurodevelopmental treatment approach and patterning have been described. The professional literature available on cerebral palsy often refers to various other approaches that have been or are still being used. Their use often depends upon the orientation and training of the professional personnel at a particular center or the philosophy of the center itself. Parents may find that physicians and therapists prefer to use a combination of approaches that best suit the developmental needs of the child.

You may hear and read about treatment techniques attributed to Phelps, Deaver, Kabat-Knott, Rood, Denhoff, and Levitt. Each has made a meaningful contribution to the comprehensive care of children with cerebral palsy. Bleck (1982) offers a fine review of various treatment techniques in the chapter on cerebral palsy in the publication "Physically Handicapped Children, a Medical Atlas for Teachers".

To learn more about the different approaches, talk with professional personnel at the treatment facility following your child. But remember, the total care and management of the child must be considered. Very likely, a comprehensive plan will include many related services and support systems.

Where Do I Obtain Additional Therapies for Home at No Cost?

More therapy at home is not necessarily the best approach to treatment for the child with cerebral palsy. This should be discussed openly with the professional personnel working with your child.

As to costs for home therapy, this will vary considerably. You may find a health department or voluntary agency that has some form of home visiting service, but it may not be on a consistently scheduled basis. You usually will find that there is a sliding-scale fee schedule for such services.

How Do I Obtain Special Equipment for Feeding and Dressing Activities?

Before you rush out to buy anything on the market, be sure that it is applicable for your child. The use of special equipment should be discussed with the members of the team working with your particular child. The physical or occupational therapist would be most knowledgeable about special items.

There are various publications that describe useful equipment for disabled persons. Such information may be available through your treatment center or from the local public library.

You may be interested in:

Functional Aids for the Multiply Handicapped by Isabel Robinault. Harper & Row Publishers, New York, 1973.

"How To's" on Dressing and Feeding (Reprinted from the book, *Handling the Young Cerebral Palsied Child at Home.*) Available from the United Cerebral Palsy Associations, New York, N.Y.

Will My Child Ever Use His Paralyzed Hand?

Observation of many children with spastic involvement of the hand and wrist demonstrates that it is possible to use the affected hand as a "helper" in most cases. Due to the nature of spasticity, it is most unlikely that the hand will be able to function fully with precise movements of the fingers.

The child should be taught to make every attempt to use the hand. There are many examples of how one hand helps the other, such as in writing. The hand affected by cerebral palsy rests on the paper while the writing is done with a pen or pencil in the better functioning hand.

Fine, intricate, and well-coordinated movements may not be possible but gross movements involving the affected hand can be accomplished. Work closely with an occupational therapist in determining the methods for obtaining optimal function of hands affected by cerebral palsy.

What Do Therapists Mean When They Refer to "ADL"?

ADL refers to the Activities of Daily Living, such as dressing, feeding, and toileting. It is a term used throughout rehabilitation and not necessarily limited to children and adults with developmental disabilities.

Usually, the activities are those that should be performed for independent living as the life situation requires. Therefore, transportation, budgeting, cooking, and laundering are some of the areas included on an as-needed basis.

ADL will be the concern of the whole rehabilitation team, with the occupational therapist giving it special emphasis.

Is Special Equipment Available for Persons with Cerebral Palsy?

There are many commercial firms that make and offer all types of special equipment to aid anyone with a disability.

Check with your treatment center's staff before sending for a catalog. Such publications usually are available in every therapy department. Some of the commercial firms prefer to have you order through a treatment center or may have a minimum required order.

There are many companies in business. Some of these advertise in special publications on the handicap as listed on page 103.

Listed below are just a few such companies:

CLEO Living Aids
3957 Mayfield Rd.
Cleveland, OH 44121

Maddak, Inc.
Pequannock, NJ 07440

J. A. Preston Corp.
60 Page Rd.
Clifton, NJ 07012

Fred Sammons, Inc.
Box 32
Brookfield, IL 60513

G. E. Miller, Inc.
484 South Broadway
Yonkers, NY 10705

Possum, Inc.
Controls for the Severely Disabled
105 Madison Ave.
New York, NY 10016

Hausmann Industries, Inc.
130 Union St.
Northvale, NJ 07647

Medco Surgical Supply
220-30 Jamaica Ave.
Queens Village, NY 11428

A word of caution: check with the therapy team to decide between variations of a product in order to select what is most useful for the person for whom it is intended.

What Is the Basis for Speech Problems?

Speech involves the uttering of vocal sounds conveying ideas. Speech problems may arise due to difficulties and problems in various areas such as intelligence, motor deficiencies of the tongue, paralysis of facial, laryngeal, or respiratory muscles, as well as the lack of social interaction.

Children with cerebral palsy may have a wide range of speech and communication difficulties. Approximately 65% of persons with cerebral palsy have some degree of difficulty with speech. The problem is determined by the extent of the brain damage, the area in which the damage occurred, and the type of cerebral palsy.

As part of the concern for a speech problem, attention should be given to auditory testing to determine how well the child hears. As with other assessment tools, such testing should be done early in order to help the child overcome special communication problems. This will be an area of concern for the speech therapist and speech pathologist on the rehabilitation team with their major efforts concentrated on treating the defective speech and developing a useful form of communication for the child and adult with cerebral palsy.

A helpful book you may want to obtain is *Cerebral Palsy and Communication,* edited by Arlene Golbin. The cost is $7.00 and the book is available from The George Washington University, Job Development Laboratory, 420 Ross Hall, 2300 Eye Street N.W., Washington, D.C. 20037.

Will My Child Ever Talk?

Perhaps it would be better if parents ask, "Will our child be able to communicate?" If the speech center in the brain is damaged, it may not be possible for the child to ever accomplish normal or intelligible speech.

A major approach to speech therapy with the child with cerebral palsy recognizes that more than just the organs of speech may be problematic in children with cerebral palsy.

Those with articulation or a spoken sound are often affected by the general problem of lack of coordination. Because of the total involvement, speech may be very difficult, often delayed, and most likely unintelligible. Treatment will depend upon a combination of approaches to the problems of articulation, breathing, facial expressions, voice control, and relaxation.

You must also consider facial expressions and gestures. If you as parents look to communication rather than just "speech" there are a variety of techniques, appliances, and special equipment that will allow even the most severely involved child with cerebral palsy to communicate with others. Intellectual ability is also important.

Working with the speech therapist and pathologist, together with other members of the professional team, you will find what is most appropriate for your child.

Can Children and Adults with Cerebral Palsy Use a Speech Synthesizer?

The synthesizer is a useful device for persons who are completely speechless or have unintelligible speech but do understand language. As an electronic device, it generates speech by either playing recorded speech segments or by synthesizing speech segments. Controlled by a built-in keyboard or switching mechanism, present equipment can hold up to 999 words, letters, or short phrases.

The unit is portable and often carried on a lap board attached to a wheelchair for severely handicapped children or adults with cerebral palsy.

A synthesizer may offer a major means of communication and lessen the frustration of the person with cerebral palsy who has the intellectual ability to use it. Physically, it does not take much to operate, usually just a touch of a finger.

It may be necessary to try different pieces of equipment before finding the one most suitable for a particular individual. Here again, involve members of the speech therapy department in a treatment setting on how best to use such equipment.

What Is "Blissymbolics"?

Blissymbolics is a combination of a picture and idea system that can be read in all languages. Through the use of approximately 100 pictures, each representing a particular idea, a person can understand a message.

When the Blissymbols are used on communication boards or electronic displays, they can be understood by observers. Originally used as a symbol system for non-speaking physically handicapped children, the concept is now being expanded for all types of disabled individuals.

Materials for teaching Blissymbolics are distributed through the Blissymbolic Communication Institute in Toronto, Canada.

If you are interested in using this material, meet with your speech therapist, who will be able to guide you on the best approach for establishing communication skills in your child.

Can a Drooling Problem Be Corrected?

Drooling in children with cerebral palsy may be due to such factors as poor control of swallowing, muscle weakness around the mouth, poor head balance, lack of sensation in the lip area, and incoordination.

Drooling is a problem for a high proportion of children with cerebral palsy and has social, educational, and hygienic implications (Harris and Dignam, 1980).

In most treatment facilities, you will find the speech therapist and occupational therapist are the professionals primarily involved in trying to correct the drooling problems. The use of biofeedback and other reward and conditioning systems are approaches to working with the child. Another technique involves the developing of an automatic response to the command "suck and swallow".

Success in overcoming the problem of drooling will vary with every child. It is a long-term program.

How Will Biofeedback Be Used in the Treatment of Children with Cerebral Palsy?

Biofeedback involves the application of external feedback of information of biological function to enable patients to alter body functions. For the child with cerebral palsy, biofeedback is just one of the innovative therapies used to get information through to the child by external means. It could involve the use of elaborate electronic equipment or more simple means of "operant conditioning."

Much remains to be done with biofeedback and children with cerebral palsy. Although there is an increasing body of knowledge describing how to use electronic devices to provide feedback information to the child with cerebral palsy, there is little information concerning how to organize, implement, and deliver this technology in an already existing treatment setting (Block and Silverstein, 1978).

Hopefully, the application of biofeedback techniques to the child with cerebral palsy will enhance the child's intelligence by allowing for greater and more effective interaction with the environment.

How Do I Obtain a List of Camps for Handicapped Children?

The most complete listing of camps for handicapped children is available from:

American Camping Association,
Bradford Woods
Martinsville, IN 46151
Ask for the Directory of Camping for the Handicapped.

The Easter Seal Society for Crippled Children and Adults has two excellent publications on camping:

1. Easter Seal Directory of Resident Camps for Persons with Special Health Needs
2. Easter Seal Guide to Special Camping Programs

Write the Society at 2023 West Ogden Avenue, Chicago, Ill. 60612.

Are There Special Playthings for Children with Cerebral Palsy?

Yes. There are many commercial firms that have special items that could be beneficial to the child with cerebral palsy or other disabled children. Although you may prefer to discuss the use of such developmental material with your therapists, you can also obtain information and catalogs by writing directly to various firms. Listed below are just a few possibilities:

> Achievement Products, Inc.
> P.O. Box 547
> Mineola, NY 11501

> Equipment Shop, Inc.
> P.O. Box 33
> Bedford, MA 01730

> Rifton Equipment
> Division of Community Playthings
> Rifton, NY 12471

> Skill Developmental Equipment Co.
> 1340 N. Jefferson St.
> P.O. Box 6300
> Anaheim, CA 92806

Is There a Listing of Special Facilities for Persons with Cerebral Palsy?

The most complete directory of all types of facilities, including educational and residential, for all types of children with disabilities, is a publication by the Porter-Sargent Publishers.

Check with your local library or treatment facility for: *The Directory for Exceptional Children: A Listing of Education and Training Facilities* edited by Ann A. Humebaugh et al. Available for $27.00 from:

> Porter-Sargent Publishers
> 11 Beacon St.
> Boston, MA 02108

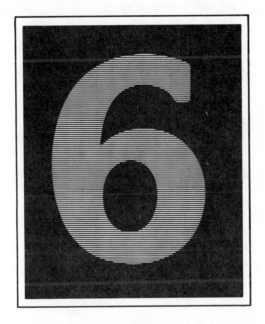

PSYCHOLOGICAL AND SOCIAL CONCERNS

Do Parents Ever Learn to Accept the Fact That They Have a Child with Cerebral Palsy?

Accepting the child with cerebral palsy as a part of the family may come slowly, but it is necessary if a normal home life is to be maintained. Many professional persons have written about the social and psychological impact of having a child with cerebral palsy and the impact on the entire family. However, this author recently read a moving article by the mother of a 7-year-old severely involved son with cerebral palsy that tells it as it is. Following correspondence with Mrs. Johann Wentzel of Roodepoort, South Africa, permission was granted to use part of the article, which first appeared in the December 1981 bulletin of the International Cerebral Palsy Society, London:

> We realised that accepting the fact that you had a handicapped child in the family was but the first milestone for the parents. To us the next important step on the road to a normal family life was to accept the way we felt from time to time. We realised how important it is to say I'm tired, I am sad, I feel helpless, I am for the moment at the end of the road, I need support.
>
> It really meant to accept your child and his handicap, your feelings about it and to accept that there are certain things one can change but there are certain things that will never be changed.
>
> We decided on a policy of complete truth, but truth with kindness. In other words we never try to give Werner false hope, but we try to motivate him to use his potential to the full.
>
> This I think is the most important decision parents have to make: what is my child's potential and how can I develop it, and what are his limitations and how do I handle that. The handicapped child is not the only person in a household whose potential should be developed. The other members of the family should be given an equal opportunity to develop their potential which might at stages be at cost of opportunity of the handicapped child. Again the answer lies in looking objectively and maintaining a fine balance.

The families should make a priority list and decide what their priorities are concerning the different members of the family. We felt that way, Werner became more part of the family and could not be blamed by the other members of the family.

We realised very clearly that we had to make changes to our life and lifestyle. But because living is giving and taking we have to give and take and so does Werner have to. If he can't go on a holiday trip, we leave him with his grandparents and the rest of the family go alone, otherwise we go during the week when he is at boarding school anyway. Our motto in coping with Werner's disability physically and emotionally is: "Accept one thing at a time. Never turn a blind eye at the future." We realised very early what is a solution today, might not be a solution tomorrow. One has to adapt to the needs of the handicapped child and to the needs of the members of the family.

This is how Johann and I learned to cope with having a handicapped child.

TESTING INTELLIGENCE

Is There Really a Way to Test the Intelligence of the Child with Cerebral Palsy?

Testing the child with cerebral palsy to determine his intellectual capabilities requires a special skill on the part of the examiner and a familiarity with several testing procedures.

For the retarded, multiply handicapped child with cerebral palsy, the usual standardized intelligence tests (such as the Stanford-Binet Intelligence Scale) are of little value because of deficits in the verbal and motor area for this population (Krasner and Silverstein, 1976).

If the testing procedure emphasizes motor skills, you will have a developmental quotient rather than an intelligence quotient. The child with cerebral palsy may do poorly in motor skills before 2 years of age and thereafter improve in the developmental quotient once verbal skills have been developed. Results can be misleading in the very young child who is not able to communicate verbally.

Properly administered, certain nonverbal tests such as the Vineland Social Maturity Scale, the Quick Test (an updated version of the picture vocabulary test), and the Griffiths Mental Developmental Scale, to mention just a few, can be used in testing the intelligence of children with cerebral palsy.

Testing children with cerebral palsy is an involved procedure. Testing should occur over a period of time. Many factors must be taken into consideration when the child is undergoing testing, such as the child's attention span, the sensory or motor capacities interfering with testing, means of communication, receptive understanding, presence of any perceptual problems, verbal and performance levels, and personality characteristics.

With specialists available for testing multiply handicapped children and the use of a variety of tests given at different periods in the child's age span, a true picture of the child's intelligence should be obtained.

To Whom Can a Parent Turn for Information?

Very often parents find their immediate family and friends do not fully understand the problems of raising a child with cerebral palsy. Although parents may feel comfortable talking with a physician about medical problems, the day-to-day situations of coping with the child with cerebral palsy may best be discussed with a professional trained to provide individual counseling. This usually is the social worker or psychologist. When necessary, such professionals will bring in other members of the treatment or educational team for assistance.

Parents will also find participating in group meetings with other parents of handicapped children a good source of support. Parent rap-groups are usually organized by the agency serving the handicapped in your area.

Another important source may be your religious affiliation. Pastoral counseling for the handicapped and their families is a concern of the clergy.

FAMILY AWARENESS

How Do You Make Family Members Aware That Cerebral Palsy Is a Permanent Condition?

Many parents indicate that relatives such as aunts and uncles and grandparents seem to think cerebral palsy is just a weakness in the child, and it will disappear. Parents hear this time and time again. No doubt the relatives mean well but have little understanding of what cerebral palsy involves. Grandparents show great concern and will find it difficult to accept the situation. Relatives may be concerned about protecting the child from the difficulties anticipated in social acceptance. There may be feelings that heredity was involved causing a nonwillingness to accept the facts of cerebral palsy. If the parents understand where the concerns are coming from, they could be more helpful in having relatives accept the child.

It is important that you as parents try to make the relatives understand that cerebral palsy will affect the child as a long-term condition. It may be helpful to involve some of the relatives in rap sessions. If feasible, grandparents should be urged to observe treatment programs with children who have cerebral palsy.

Opportunities to talk with professional personnel should be made available. As part of the long-range planning for the child with cerebral palsy, relatives need to realize that a family having a child with cerebral palsy must have complete understanding and support.

What, If Anything, Can Be Done So That People Will Better Understand and Not Shun the Individual with Cerebral Palsy?

Much has been done . . . much is being done . . . and much still needs to be done.

Ongoing campaigns by private and governmental agencies are geared to bring about a better understanding of the abilities of the handicapped. In particular, with cerebral palsy, public relations through the various media, especially TV, have been instrumental in making the general public aware of the term *cerebral palsy*. Whether or not one agrees that children and adults with cerebral palsy should not be seen on nationally televised telethons, public awareness has been accomplished.

Full acceptance of the child or adult with cerebral palsy is still the goal for parents and professionals. It will not happen overnight.

Every effort must be made to continue educating the public about *all* handicapped people. Parents have a very special role to play. They can do much by reaching into the community and telling the story of cerebral palsy. The United Cerebral Palsy Associations is truly an example of what can be accomplished when a handful of parents decide that something can be done to bring about a better understanding of persons with cerebral palsy.

Why Do Some Professional Personnel Feel That the Parents Are Not Capable of Understanding Hard Facts?

Much has been written about the attitudes of professional personnel in different situations. You may meet parents who express concern about the lack of information given to them in response to specific questions. This could be interpretation of information on the part of the parent. Many parents indicate they were not willing or ready to accept certain information offered by professional personnel. Occasionally, the professional person with whom you come in contact may appear to be withholding information. This may be due to the professional's concern that the parent is not ready to accept information at a particular time.

When a good relationship has been established between parent and the professional worker, there is little need for either party to withhold information. You both need trust! If at any time you as a parent feel "hard facts" are not being discussed, raise the question with your professional contact. You may be dealing with differences of opinion and it is best to keep all information out in the open. This will allow for a better working and trusting relationship to be established. There is no need for either party to withhold information or to omit constructive discussion of remaining options.

Can We Expect Feelings of Jealousy from Other Children in the Family?

Many studies have demonstrated that sibling jealousy or rivalry is quite likely to occur in a family with a handicapped child.

A study completed in England with mothers who had at least one other child in the family found that 33% of the mothers reported sibling jealousy of the child's handicapped brother or sister. In his book, *Handicap and Family Crisis,* Stephen Kew (1975) suggests that any figures reported in different studies tend to underestimate the extent of the problem.

To many parents, the amount of time devoted to the care of the handicapped child creates a problem of sharing time with all the children. Some families cope with this situation very well by being sure that the child with the handicap is treated as normally as possible.

If the child with cerebral palsy is only mildly affected, it becomes easier for the parents to handle all situations in a normal atmosphere at home. The more severely handicapped children with cerebral palsy do require a great deal of attention from parents, thus opening the possibilities of unintentional neglect of other siblings. The situation is subject to change as the needs of the child with cerebral palsy become ever increasingly evident.

Sibling rivalry and jealousy can be a real problem to the family of a handicapped child. Parents and siblings should feel free to discuss any such problems with professional personnel such as the psychologist or social worker, who should be able to offer appropriate guidance.

Does the Size of the Family
Affect the Child with Cerebral Palsy?

There seems to be no clear evidence that a child with cerebral palsy is better off in a large family or in a small family.

In the literature on handicapped children, it is often suggested that a handicapped child in a large family stands a chance of getting a lot of attention from many people. Parents have often expressed the feeling that having several brothers and sisters made for a more normal environment in which everyone took part of the responsibility in caring for the child with cerebral palsy. On the other hand, having a large family may mean less parental time for each child.

The child with cerebral palsy in a small family of one or two other children may require much more care than the others, which in turn could develop into sibling problems. Parents of an only child with cerebral palsy stand the risk of devoting every moment of their life to the care of that child. Such parents also speak of marital problems because of disagreements that arise in the approach to handling the handicapped child.

Despite all that may occur with a child in a small or large family, most families manage to raise the handicapped child without serious incident. Let no one tell you how to plan your family. This is your decision!

Will Our Other Children Be Concerned
about Bringing Their Friends into Our Home?

This question, often asked by parents, really is "Will my son be embarrassed to bring his girlfriend into my house?" or "Will my daughter be reluctant to bring her boyfriend home?" Parents are concerned that siblings will react negatively and go through an emotional crisis when it comes to having the child with cerebral palsy at home seen by others. The attitudes developed by brothers and sisters will depend primarily on how the family has accepted the handicapped child throughout the years.

In some families, there are siblings who completely reject the handicapped child and do not care to have friends involved in their family situation. Socially, the sibling may feel he or she would be rejected by friends when they see a handicapped brother or sister at home. This may be due to an attitude that has been developed by society in general and not necessarily a demonstration of dislike among siblings.

To overcome some of the sibling problems, parents themselves have indicated every attempt should be made to involve friends of the siblings in the activities of the home. Siblings often need help in understanding the situation when they enter the adolescent period. This may happen despite the fact that parents have provided a happy, secure home for all the children.

Siblings should be made aware of the causes of cerebral palsy, beginning with simple explanations when they are young. More information should be made available as they grow older. They should have knowledge and practice in explaining their disabled family member to others throughout the years. If the cause of the condition is known, this should be shared with the siblings.

Siblings should also be made aware of future plans for the child with cerebral palsy. This may allay any fears that they will have to be responsible for caring for the disabled person.

It may also be necessary to reassure friends of the siblings that cerebral palsy is not a disease and is nonprogressive. The more information made available to friends of the siblings the greater the acceptance of the handicapped child will be.

SPECIAL ACTIVITIES

Is There a Resource List That Tells Parents Where They Can Get Information on Various Programs, Special Activities, and Financial Aid?

There are many resources available to the parents of a child with cerebral palsy, but they may not find them all in one place.

Start by asking your local community service agency for a directory of services. Usually the community or the state education department or social service agency maintains a directory which lists all public, private, and governmental agencies serving the area. You may find what you want under such headings as handicapped, disabled, rehabilitation, special education, vocational training, health care, recreation, welfare, or cerebral palsy.

You may also find it to your advantage to participate in the activities of your area organization devoted to serving persons with cerebral palsy. Such an organization will most likely have a newsletter with information about local programming. You should also place your name on the mailing lists of state or national groups serving the cerebral palsied. Newsletters will help you keep up with the most recent advances in research and treatment as well as other practical information.

It is most important that the parents of the young child with cerebral palsy try to become active members and participants in the activities of the educational and treatment facilities their child attends.

Among the national organizations that stand ready to assist parents of children and adults with cerebral palsy are:

United Cerebral Palsy Associations, Inc.
66 West 34 Street
New York, NY 10016

Association for Retarded Citizens
P.O. Box 6109
Arlington, TX 76011

Epilepsy Foundation of America
4351 Garden City Drive
Landover, MD 20785

National Easter Seal Society
2023 West Ogden
Chicago, IL 60612

Where Are Parents Left When Doctors Say They Know Very Little About Cerebral Palsy?

This may be a matter of interpretation. When the physician or any other professional person indicates little is known about cerebral palsy, this may refer to the long range effects of the overall condition.

A great amount of information about the causes, prevention, treatment, and characteristics of cerebral palsy is known. The major problem that arises is that every child and adult with cerebral palsy is different. There are so many possible influences on the development of the child with cerebral palsy that can affect the future of that person. These influences make it most difficult for anyone to state, beyond doubt, what the outcome of the condition will be.

To help the child to reach full potential, it may be necessary to establish short-term, realistic goals. Parents must remain hopeful and realistic, knowing that what information is available about cerebral palsy is applicable to meet the specific needs of any child.

What Does the Term "Shopping Parents" Mean?

When first made aware that their child has cerebral palsy, many parents are not able to accept the diagnosis. Parents may feel it is absolutely necessary to go to various professional (and nonprofessional) people, hoping to have someone say the child has a less serious condition. Such searching, or *shopping,* was quite in order in the early 1940s and 1950s as the ability to identify the condition of cerebral palsy was limited to far fewer specialists than today.

With the type of diagnostic services and early intervention programs available today, one should see a lessening for the need to shop for help and assistance.

There is no doubt that you still will hear of parents who are not willing to accept the fact that their child is less than perfect. Much valuable time, energy, and money may be spent in shopping when all efforts should be directed toward programming for the child.

Be cautious about continuing to look for that one person who will tell you what you want to hear!

Do All People with Cerebral Palsy Develop Unusual Personality Traits?

Many studies have been conducted indicating there is little relationship between the kind of handicap or disability and one's personality.

You cannot generalize by saying a person with cerebral palsy has a "cerebral palsy personality." Every person has his or her own personality and we all differ in many ways. What is appropriate for the nondisabled population applies equally as well to those persons with cerebral palsy.

How and When Should We Explain to Our Child What He or She Has and How It Happened?

If your child has a good understanding of what is going on in the immediate environment, he or she will recognize that a difference does exist in their relationships with other people.

Children with cerebral palsy need to be made aware of their condition from the time the first question is asked. Responses may be simple at first, progressing in complexity and factual data as the child grows and is able to understand more. The child will also find answers to his or her problems as new experiences are offered.

Parents often indicate that, despite the amount of knowledge and information they have on cerebral palsy, they have found it difficult to explain to their child. However, parents should not underestimate how much the child learns about the condition from participation in special educational and treatment programs.

Those children with cerebral palsy who have limited intellectual capacity may never need a thorough explanation on its causes and effects.

What Can Be Done When Parents Blame Their Child for Being Cerebral Palsied?

Such a situation calls for psychological support for the parents. If the parents are involved in the treatment services offered by their local health facility, counseling may be available from a psychologist or social worker. If such staff is not available, arrangements usually can be made for counseling from other local sources, such as a hospital, private practitioner, or social service program.

Counseling plays a very important role in bringing about the understanding of the parents and the child. If attention is not given to the problem of nonacceptance of the child, further consequences may develop that will interfere with the total management of the child with cerebral palsy.

Parents should recognize that counseling or psychotherapy is a supportive measure and may be considered a necessary part of the treatment program planned for the child and the family.

During therapy sessions, the treatment center staff may observe problems of nonacceptance of the child. These problems may be demonstrated by a parent's lack of interest or poor attitude. A referral for counseling may be appropriate at that time.

What Happens When the Child Blames the Parents for His or Her Having Cerebral Palsy?

It is very likely that a child who is intellectually high functioning will react negatively to parents by blaming them for his or her having cerebral palsy. At some time in almost every child's life the words *I hate you* may be spoken. This can happen with the child with cerebral palsy as well. In particular, the disabled child who has a good understanding of the social implications of being handicapped may develop a very negative attitude toward the parents.

Appropriate psychological counseling should be sought before feelings interfere with the total social maturation process. Seek out the psychologist or social worker at your treatment facility before the problem becomes overwhelming and a major disturbing influence in the home.

In Caring for a Child with Cerebral Palsy, What Expenses Are Deductible?

Many of the expenses incurred by parents of any disabled child are subject to tax deductions. These may apply to medical care, special services, special aids, transportation, medical insurance, and therapeutic activities.

Check with your local Internal Revenue Service if you have any questions. A well-versed accountant familiar with all the possible tax credits and deductions is vital.

A nine-page article, "Annual Income Tax Guide" that appeared in the December 1981 issue (Vol. 11 No. 6) of the Exceptional Parent magazine would be most worthwhile reading. Contact the magazine at:

> Exceptional Parent
> 296 Boylston St.
> Boston, MA 02116

COMMUNITY SERVICES

Do Persons with Cerebral Palsy Have a Right to Community Services?

Cerebral palsy is included in the definition of "developmental disabilities." According to the legal department of the United Cerebral Palsy Associations (Neuwirth, 1980), the United States Third Circuit Court of Appeals handed down a decision in the *Halderman* vs. *Pennhurst State School and Hospital,* December 13, 1979. The 6-to-3 ruling is a declaration that:

...all developmentally disabled people are entitled to education, training and care to reach their maximum development

...such habilitative services must be provided in the least restrictive setting

...there are strong legislative presumptions that community settings, not institutions, are the appropriate places for habilitation of all retarded and developmentally disabled persons

What Can I Do as a Parent Politically?

Parents can play a very important role in seeking and in supporting legislation for the handicapped. Every legislator knows there may be at least two votes in the household. If you cannot participate in demonstrations or make trips to your legislator, you can still do a lot behind the scenes.

Gil Joel (1975) in his book, *So Your Child Has Cerebral Palsy,* indicates "that parents of the cerebral palsied are conspicuous by their absence in any expression of political action, be it demonstration or letter writing." He points out that involvement in such activities will not only help your child and others but may open new interests for the parents that may go well beyond the original concern.

It is advisable to try to work with other parents or your cerebral palsy association. Together the parents have a strong voice, one that legislators will listen to.

How Does a Parent Find Out
What Recreational Activities Are Available
for the Child or Adult with Cerebral Palsy?

Space limitations make it impossible to list all of the organizations in the country that offer special programs for the child or adult with cerebral palsy.

Generally, it is the philosophy of many health agencies to go beyond the concept of treatment by offering programs that include recreation. Some of these may be day camping, travel, weekend outings, scouting, swimming, summer camping, and all types of planned recreation.

If there is a United Cerebral Palsy Association or an Easter Seal Society in your community, seek them out. A call to the local United Fund organization for a listing of participating agencies will also give you a good idea of what is available.

Recreation is an important part of learning and provides many opportunities for socialization. Seek out the programs! And if resources are limited, get a few people together and start something.

How Will I Manage Air Travel
with My Child with Cerebral Palsy?

The Federal Aviation Administration has issued a guidebook aimed at making air travel easier and more convenient for the handicapped and elderly persons.

The publication lists design features of airports, facilities, and services that meet the travel needs of the wheelchair bound, the blind, and the deaf. The latest edition includes information on 282 airport terminals in 40 countries. For each terminal, the guide identifies 70 features important to handicapped travelers, including reserved parking, ramps, accessible rest rooms, elevator controls, telephones, and special transportation.

Single copies of the guide are free. Ask for:

Access Travel: Airports
Architectural and Transportation Barriers
   Compliance Board
330 C St. S.W.
Washington, DC 20201

What Can Be Done to Help the Person with Cerebral Palsy Have a Better Social Life?

Participating in social activities can be a real problem for many persons with cerebral palsy. If the individual is severely handicapped and has the intellectual capacity to enjoy other people's company, there may be some very frustrating times ahead. Social activities will depend on how well the disabled person can be integrated into various groups. For those persons with cerebral palsy involved in an active program sponsored by one of the many voluntary agencies working with the handicapped, there could be many opportunities for socialization. As the child with cerebral palsy matures, however, you may find less opportunities for socialization, especially with the nondisabled population.

Despite all of the advances made in trying to bring about a better understanding of the disabled, it is rare to see a group of nonhandicapped teenagers socializing with a classmate who is cerebral palsied. This is especially so if the person with cerebral palsy is severely handicapped and in need of assistance.

The mildly involved child or young adult with cerebral palsy (and good intellect) may easily be accepted into a peer group. This is especially so if the person with cerebral palsy has attended a regular school and his classmates are true friends.

A parent may have to establish the climate for socialization by making the home the center of activities so that classmates will want to be with the disabled child. The frustration will come in the adolescent years when companionship is needed and difficult to find. Camps, scouting, recreation, or interest groups may offer some options.

Does It Help If a Person with Cerebral Palsy Gets Involved with Politics?

Being involved in politics may be just what is needed to bring about certain changes on behalf of the handicapped.

A person with cerebral palsy should be able to participate in various political activities including lobbying for legislation. Only recently have disabled people banded together to make legislative leaders aware of their needs. There have been sit-ins at federal offices and meetings with legislators. Many of the changes that have resulted in the elimination of architectural barriers have been the result of the political activism of a small group of people with disabilities.

People with cerebral palsy may not always be able to "march to the capitol" but they can work on letter writing campaigns, make phone calls, support an assembly of handicapped people by their very presence, and appear before legislative hearings.

It takes involvement! If the adult with cerebral palsy has any inclination toward such involvement in the political arena, it should be encouraged.

For further information contact:

Advocacy Coordinator
United Cerebral Palsy Associations, Inc.
66 East 34 St.
New York, NY 10016

Are There Any Periodicals Geared to Meet the Needs of Parents of Children or Adults with Cerebral Palsy?

There are several publications that include information of all types that certainly would be of interest to parents of children or adults with cerebral palsy.

The Exceptional Parent, a magazine published in Boston, is one of the best sources of information for parents of children and adults with all types of problems. Circulation of the magazine is approximately 20,000 readers. It is published six times a year. Subscription for 1 year is $15, for 2 years $28, and for 3 years $39. Write:

> The Exceptional Parent
> 296 Boylston St. (Third Floor)
> Boston, MA 02116

The Bridge will research and report on all aspects of living and services available for the handicapped. Issued monthly. The cost is $10 for 12 issues. Write:

> The Bridge
> Beecher House, Inc.
> P.O. Box 1253
> Madison, CT 06443

Accent on Living is published quarterly and offers information on new products for the disabled and interesting information on available services. Subscription rate is $4 for 1 year; $7.25 for 2 years; and $10.50 for 3 years. Write:

> Accent on Living
> Cheever Publishing, Inc.
> P.O. Box 700
> Gillum Rd. and High Dr.
> Bloomington, IL 61701

Up Front is a newspaper for handicapped and disabled persons, published 11 times a year. Subscription rates are $15 for 1 year and $25 for 2 years. Write:

> Up Front
> 55 West Park Ave.
> New Haven, CT 06511

Rehabilitation Gazette is published yearly. This international journal on independent living written by disabled persons for disabled people covers lifestyles, special equipment, resources and coping skills. Donation per copy is $4.50 from disabled individuals and $7 from the public at large. Write:

> *Rehabilitation Gazette*
> 4502 Maryland Ave.
> St. Louis, MO 63108

How Can I Get Information on Special Programs Throughout the Country?

One of the major sources for information on services is:

> Closer Look Parent's Campaign for
>   Handicapped Children and Youth
> P.O. Box 1492
> Washington, DC 20013

Closer Look has all types of information on many different service programs located throughout the country and can serve as an excellent resource for parents in need of information.

If, as a parent of a child or adult with cerebral palsy, you are affiliated with a United Cerebral Palsy Association, the local organization will be able to help you. There is a well-established network of United Cerebral Palsy affiliates throughout the country. All types of information is available through the local, state, or national offices.

What Can We Do as Parents to Assist Our Child in an Ultimate Goal of Independence As an Adult?

The obvious response to this question is to allow the child to develop all the capabilities he or she may have. This will not be an easy task. There will be many times that you as parents will feel the need to overprotect the child. There will also be times when you recognize that the child must do certain things on his or her own.

Parents do not have to do the whole job all by themselves. Most important is having the ability to search out available resources in the community and be sure they are used to the best advantage of your child and family.

One parent who replied to this author's request for questions had "one million other questions, but my son has not gotten as far as he has by my asking questions, but by putting my energies to work dealing with what I had and making what he had work to the best of his abilities. . . and then some."

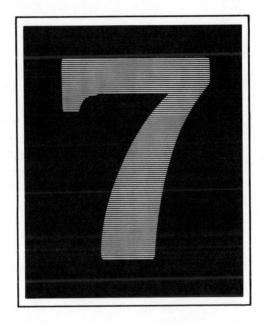

EDUCATIONAL
CONCERNS

PUBLIC LAW 94-142

What Is Public Law 94-142?

Enacted in 1976, Public Law 94-142 is the Education for All Handicapped Children Act. The law declares education a fundamental right that must be extended to all handicapped individuals. It provides for a free education plus certain related services when indicated for handicapped people between the ages of 3 and 21.

It should be noted that the responsibility for the education of all handicapped children rests with the proper educational agency in the state.

For information on the rights of disabled children and general material on public education, write:

Closer Look Information Center
1201 16th Street N.W.
Washington, DC 20036

Is Cerebral Palsy Specifically Included in Public Law 94-142?

It is not necessary for the actual term *cerebral palsy* to be specifically written into the law.

Handicapped children means those evaluated as being mentally retarded, hard of hearing, deaf, speech impaired, visually handicapped, seriously emotionally disturbed, orthopedically impaired, otherwise health impaired, deaf-blind, multi-handicapped, or as having specific learning disabilities, who because of these impairments need special education and related services. Each is specifically defined in the federal regulations in Section 121 a.5.

When Must a School System Provide Education to a Handicapped Child?

Public Law 94-142 took effect October 1, 1977. At that time school systems were to meet the law's provisions with respect to identifying handicapped children, writing IEPs, and enrolling handicapped children, but they could legally provide less than a free appropriate public education.

As of September 1, 1978, a free appropriate public education must be provided to all handicapped children age 3 through 18 and as of September 1, 1980, for all handicapped children age 3 through 21. Schools are not necessarily legally bound to provide education for handicapped children age 3 to 5 and 18 through 21 if such education is inconsistent with state law or practice or any court order.

The general rule is that whenever education is provided for nonhandicapped children of these ages, it must also be available to handicapped children.

Under Public Law 94-142, there are special incentive grants available to encourage school systems to provide special education to handicapped children at ages 3, 4, and 5.

What Are the Parent's Rights Under the Law?

Parents of handicapped children must be notified in writing before a public agency initiates, changes, or refuses to initiate or change the identification, evaluation, or placement of the child or the provision of a free appropriate public education to the child. This notification in the parents' native language or other mode of communication (braille, oral communication, sign language) must include:

1. A full explanation of parents' due process rights
2. A description of the action proposed or refused by the agency, why the agency proposes or refuses to take this action, and a description of any options considered by the agency and reasons why they were rejected
3. A description of each evaluation procedure, test, record, or report the agency uses as a basis for the proposal or refusal
4. Any other factors relevant to the agency's proposal or refusal.

What Is Meant by the Term
Free and Appropriate Public Education?

Free and appropriate public education means special education and related services provided at the preschool, elementary, or secondary education level. These must be at public expense and under public supervision and must meet standards of the state educational agency.

Under Public Law 94-142, each handicapped child requiring special education must have an individualized education program as evidence that he or she is receiving a free appropriate education.

How Does One Go About Getting Information on Recently Passed Legislation Outlining What Obligations the Public School Has to Handicapped Children?

If you do not wish to go about getting the information from the local school principal, administrative offices, or school district, go directly to the state education department. More specifically, write the bureau or division that services handicapped children.

Information on new legislation may also be obtained from your locally elected state legislators. They appreciate hearing from their constituents and usually have a staff to obtain the material you request.

Participation in the activities of a parent group will also give you an opportunity to hear about new programs and recently passed legislation.

Your local library should be considered an important source of information. Librarians know where to obtain information and are known to have responded to the needs of the handicapped.

What Are My Child's Rights to Special Education?

There is a simple-to-use checklist now available that parents will find useful in determining whether their schools are serving disabled children in accordance with the federal law.

Single copies of the *Special Education Checkup* are free to parents sending a stamped, self-addressed, business size envelope to:

The National Committee for Citizens in Education
Dept. SEC
410 Wilde Lake Village Green
Columbia, MD 21044

There is also a publication, *Parents Can Be the Key* that offers information on parents' rights and the education process. Advocacy and legal services are listed. The 28-page booklet is available for $1.00 from:

Pacer Center, Inc.
4701 Chicago Ave., So.
Minneapolis, MN 55407

Another informative guide, by David Lillie and Patricia Place, is *Partners: A Guide to Working with Schools for Parents of Children with Special Instructional Needs* available for $8.95 from:

Scott, Foresman and Co.
1900 East Lake Ave.
Glenview, IL 60025

How Do I Obtain Education for My Child Under Age 5?

In all states, educational services are provided for handicapped children between the ages of 5 and 21 under the provisions of federal law (the Education for All Handicapped Children Act) and applicable state law. Services for handicapped children under the age of 5 years vary in different states.

Services for the younger child may depend upon the diagnostic classification of the child, for example, hearing impaired children may start education in the preschool years.

You can obtain specific information on the rules and regulations governing education for all handicapped children by contacting the state department of education. Your local legislator should also be in the position to obtain the information for you. The school district should also be able to supply any information on education of the very young child.

Can a Child with Cerebral Palsy Participate in a Head Start Program?

Project Head Start is a child development program providing various educational and social services, parent involvement and health services to preschool children between the ages of 3 and 5, of low-income families.

In 1972, Amendments to the Economic Opportunity Act called for at least 10% of the nationwide enrollment in Head Start to consist of children who are handicapped and require special services. Therefore, children with cerebral palsy meeting the requirements would be eligible for a Head Start program.

The term *handicapped children,* as defined in the Act, includes "mentally retarded, hard of hearing, deaf, speech impaired, visually handicapped, seriously emotionally disturbed, orthopedically impaired, or other health impaired children or children with specific learning disabilities who by reason thereof require special education and related services."

For information about the Head Start program in your area, check with your local school district or look in the phone book for Project Head Start.

Will There Be Any Problems Placing a Child with Cerebral Palsy in a Regular School?

Whether or not there will be a problem placing the child with cerebral palsy into a regular school will depend on many factors.

With the concept of mainstreaming prevalent today, it is possible to place the child with cerebral palsy in regular school systems. The major question to be considered is whether or not such placement offers the most appropriate education for the child in the least restrictive setting.

The school must be willing to accept the disabled child and be prepared to offer special services. The severely handicapped child may not be well integrated into all programs a regular school has to offer, whereas a mildly involved child may have no difficulty. The parents must consider the long range benefits of placement in a regular school as compared to what the child may or may not receive in a special education program.

It has been estimated that only 10% of the children assigned to special classes are ever returned to the regular classroom. This has led many educators to demand that programs be adapted to individual learning needs and that there be regular evaluations of progress. Such an approach could result in a greater percentage of reintegration with normal classes (Rauth, 1980).

Will Most Handicapped Children
Be Placed in Regular Classrooms?

Placement must be based on each individual child's needs. If a handicapped child can learn and function in a regular classroom, such placement is required. The law recognizes, however, that not all children will benefit from the regular class environment.

Public Law 94-142 requires that a continuum of alternative placements be available including instruction in regular classes, special classes, home instruction, and instruction in hospitals and institutions. Federal regulations, in fact, require that "in selecting the least restrictive environment, consideration is given to any potential harmful effect on the child or on the quality of services he or she needs."

What Is It Like for a Child with Mild Cerebral Palsy to Be in a Regular School with Other Children?

Young adults with cerebral palsy who have attended regular schools have said there were many difficult times.

It is generally accepted that children can be cruel at times when it comes to accepting someone who is different. The child with a mild case of cerebral palsy may still need some help in routine activities or perhaps may be unable to participate fully in everything that goes on in the class. Where possible, the teacher should be made aware of any limitations the child may have and suggestions for coping with them before the child enters the school. Some teachers have found it very worthwhile to discuss the newcomer with other classmates to bring about a better understanding.

The child with cerebral palsy will no doubt recognize he or she is not completely accepted until all the other children realize that the mild handicap does not interfere with the child's being a friend. Very often, the child with cerebral palsy needs to excel in some area that draws attention and respect from others.

Your child may have a difficult time at first, but with support from understanding teachers and the family, accep- tance can be obtained. Remember, your child must grow up in a world of normal people, and the sooner the child is involved with normal children, the better he or she will be.

It is advisable for parents to watch the situation in a new classroom very carefully. Work with the teacher and others to resolve any problems that may develop.

What Happens If the School System Does Not Follow the Law?

If your school system refuses to comply with the law, the state may withhold the school system's share of federal funds under Public Law 94-142 and possibly some state funds in accordance with the provisions of state law on education of the handicapped. The state could also refuse future applications by the school system for Public Law 94-142 funds on the basis of noncompliance. Such funds can be withheld only after the local education agency has been given reasonable notice and an opportunity for a hearing.

In addition, the federal government may withhold funds for education of the handicapped from an entire state. This can be done only after reasonable notice and an opportunity for a hearing is provided. These are extreme measures! State and school systems in violation, when put on notice, usually find some way to come into compliance with the law.

What Is The Committee on the Handicapped?

Often referred to as the *COH,* the Committee on the Handicapped is a group of people who meet on a regular basis to make recommendations regarding the education of children who require special education. The recommendations are made to the local Board of Education and to the parents of the child.

The committee determines what the children need based on a review of various types of reports and evaluations.

By law each school district must have a COH. The committee itself includes the following people: a school psychologist, a teacher or administrator of special education, a physician, a parent of a handicapped child who lives in the district, and may also include other people appointed by the Board of Education. As a parent, you have the right and obligation to work closely with the committee in your district.

THE INDIVIDUALIZED EDUCATIONAL PROGRAM

What Is an IEP?

IEP refers to the Individualized Educational Program that must be developed jointly by parents and professionals in educational and treatment facilities in accordance with the federal regulations stipulated in Public Law 94-142.

The IEP details the total program that the child with a handicap, in need of special education, should receive, and includes not only educational goals but where necessary, the supportive and special services each child may require.

Developing the IEP takes a great deal of time and effort on the part of many people. The effectiveness of the IEP has yet to be determined.

How Can Parents of a Child with Cerebral Palsy Be Better Prepared for an Evaluation Team Meeting?

Parents of the child with cerebral palsy participating in a "team evaluation" meeting, conducted by school personnel, should be prepared to be a full participant in the session. The meeting, usually held before admission to school, will allow for an exchange of information between parents and professional personnel and help decide the future programming for the child. In some situations, the meeting may be considered as the same session in which the Individualized Education Program is developed. All the material that is obtained could be subject to other reviews at future dates.

To assist parents in taking an active role at such meetings, a special checklist has been prepared by the Association for Retarded Citizens, Philadelphia Chapter. Permission has been granted by the Chapter to use the material in this publication. The checklist should be reviewed and completed by parents before attending the evaluation meeting.

It should be noted that all of the items on the checklist may not pertain to every child. Choose the pertinent items for your child and your situation.

Because the checklist was developed by one organization, it is possible that terms designating various personnel or units may not apply in another area. For example, CSET refers to Child Study Evaluation Team, a term specific to the Philadelphia area and program. Your school district may use another term to refer to the evaluation team.

EVALUATION CHECKLIST

Child Study Evaluation Team (CSET) Checklist

Complete this list before attending the CSET meeting. This checklist and the "Checklist for IEP meeting" can be used jointly in the CSET meeting. All items on this checklist do not pertain to each child. Check only the items that pertain to your child.

Preparation for CSET meeting   YES   NO

I have a copy of all my child's school records.   ____ ____

Each test has been administered within a year of
    today's date. (The School District does not have   ____ ____
    to do yearly tests, but the parent can request an
    annual evaluation, in which case the School
    District must try to comply.)

If NO, I have requested a recent test of the type
    that is outdated.   ____ ____

Each of the following persons has seen my child in preparation for
    the CSET meeting. (These are core team members who should
    be involved in every CSET.)
        Educational Evaluator   ____ ____
        School Nurse   ____ ____
        Psychologist   ____ ____
        Counselor *(It is appropriate that the counselor*   ____ ____
            see parents in addition to the child.)

Each person completing a report has actually seen
    my child.   ____ ____

If NO, I have requested that the team member see
    the child prior to the CSET meeting.   ____ ____

Each of the following evaluations has been done. *(Check only
    those that you think the child needs or that one of the team
    members has recommended.)*
        Physical Therapist   ____ ____
        Psychiatrist   ____ ____
        Optometrist   ____ ____
        Neurologist   ____ ____
        Music Therapist   ____ ____
        Orthopedic Specialist   ____ ____
        Hearing Therapist or Audiologist   ____ ____
        Speech Therapist   ____ ____
        Occupational Therapist   ____ ____
        Ophthalmologist   ____ ____
        Art Therapist   ____ ____
        Movement Therapist   ____ ____

Behavior Therapist   _____ _____

Other _____ _____ _____

Check yes or no.   YES   NO

I have a copy of the present Individualized Educational Program and will review it prior to the CSET meeting. (This is important in order to establish where the child is presently functioning developmentally.) _____ _____

I have advised my Base Service Unit and/or advocate that the CSET process is beginning and have asked for their involvement. _____ _____

I have signed permission to release records for the Base Service Unit and/or advocate, who can then request records from the School District. _____ _____

The School District has requested records from other sources in order to better understand my child. _____ _____

List all the sources that I would like the School District to contact for records. (You may wish to list hospitals or clinics, educational programs that the child has previously been enrolled in, and any other agency that has dealt with your child and that you would like to forward records to the School District.)

More than one test was administered to my child to determine his/her present abilities. _____ _____

The tests that were administered to my child did not appear to me to be racially or culturally discriminatory. _____ _____

The tests were administered to my child in his/her native language. _____ _____

All records and reports were interpreted to me if they were not in my native language. _____ _____

The CSET Meeting

The core evaluators are present

Counselor _____ _____

Educational Evaluator _____ _____

School Nurse _____ _____

Psychologist _____ _____

If NO, they have submitted a written report prior to the meeting, and I have a copy of it. _____ _____

I am asked for my ideas and am given ample time to talk during this meeting. _____ _____

The principal or his/her designee is present.   _____ _____

The child's current teacher is present.   _____ _____

(This is appropriate if the child is presently in an educational program. The teacher could be from the School District or from another program such as a preschool that the child is currently attending.)

The Base Service Unit representative and/or advocate is present if I wish.   _____ _____

I have requested a copy of each of the evaluators' reports.   _____ _____

(You will probably not receive these unless you request them.)

Discussion in the meeting focuses on my child's strengths as well as weaknesses in each of the following areas:

    Communication   _____ _____
    Cognitive   _____ _____
    Gross Motor   _____ _____
    Fine Motor   _____ _____
    Social-Emotional   _____ _____
    Health and Physical   _____ _____
    Other (explain)   _____ _____

The CSET Final Report

I have requested a copy of the CSET final summary report.   _____ _____

(This is a document that summarizes suggestions and findings of all the evaluators.)

My child's strengths and weaknesses in each of the following areas are noted:

    Communication   _____ _____
    Cognitive   _____ _____
    Gross Motor   _____ _____
    Fine Motor   _____ _____
    Social-Emotional   _____ _____
    Health and Physical   _____ _____
    Other (explain)   _____ _____

I have read the CSET report and do not disagree with any of the statements in it.   _____ _____

(If I disagree with a statement, I have initiated discussion with the principal regarding my disagreement.)

I have read the CSET report and do not have any
additions to suggest.   _____ _____
*(If I note an omission, I have initiated discussion
with the principal regarding the statements that I
would like included in the report.)*
Services which should be helpful to my child are
noted in the final report.   _____ _____
I have given my permission for the principal to
release a copy of the CSET final report to my
Base Service Unit worker and/or my advocate.   _____ _____
I have discussed this report with the Base Service
Unit worker and/or advocate and have consid-
ered their suggestions.   _____ _____
*(In the event that they recommend any changes or
additions with which I agree, I have initiated dis-
cussion with the principal.)*

After the CSET report is completed, the process to develop the
Individualized Educational Program (IEP) should begin. The IEP
should be based on the findings in the CSET report, so you will
continually want to refer to the CSET report as you are giving your
suggestions for the IEP. This office has also prepared an IEP
Checklist to assist you in participating in the IEP meeting.

Anyone wishing more information about these checklists should
contact: The Association For Retarded Citizens, Philadelphia
Chapter, 1211 Chestnut Street, Philadelphia, PA 19107. Their
phone number is 215-567-3750.

Reprinted with permission of The Association for Retarded Citizens, Philadelphia Chapter.

When Must the Yearly Individual Education Program Be Developed?

An IEP must be completed for each of those handicapped children in need of special education programs by the beginning of the school year.

The IEP must be in effect before special education and related services are provided.

Is There a Checklist One Can Use in Preparation for an IEP Meeting?

Thanks to the Association for Retarded Citizens, Philadelphia Chapter, a special checklist has been prepared for use by parents planning to attend the IEP meeting. The checklist could serve as a guide to be sure that those services you as a parent want for your child are included in the final written plan.

As a suggested checklist, this material could be very helpful to parents of children with cerebral palsy.

PREPARE YOURSELF

Complete before you go to the IEP (Individualized Education Program) meeting and use as a guide for making sure those services that you want are included in the final written plan.

Does Your Child Need . . .   YES   NO

speech therapy _____ _____
physical therapy _____ _____
occupational therapy _____ _____
art _____ _____
aid in classroom _____ _____
transportation _____ _____
   if so, door to door? _____ _____
   matron on bus? _____ _____
   lift bus? _____ _____
   restraint (seat belt, etc.)? _____ _____

Should lunch be a part of instructional time?   _____ _____

(Check YES only if your child needs to learn skills that are associated with lunch, such as chewing, self-feeding.)
vocational programming   _____ _____

Does Your Child Need . . .   YES   NO

summer program   _____ _____
medication in school   _____ _____
if so, how transported? _____
if so, how given? _____
toilet training   _____ _____
psychotherapy   _____ _____
counseling   _____ _____
nurse in school   _____ _____
mobility training   _____ _____
   (help in learning how to use public transportation)
help in learning how to use leisure time   _____ _____
instruction in body awareness, functions and
   systems   _____ _____
hearing   _____ _____
a special diet   _____ _____
Will you be sending lunch to school with your
child?   _____ _____

Questions to Ask During the IEP Meeting

Ask questions about these areas during the meeting and look for information on these points before you sign the IEP.

— What is the plan for physical education? (Required for all students.)
— How many students and how many teachers and aides working directly with the students will there be in each classroom the child will be in?
— If your child is physically handicapped:
   What floor will the child's classroom(s) be on?
   Are the building(s) accessible?
   Will any special assistance be required, such as in toileting?
   Where are the bathrooms to the proposed classroom(s) located? Are they in the room or adjacent? What is the distance between the classroom(s) and toilet facilities?
— Check how many hours and where student will be in each of the following:
   —Regular classroom
   —Resource room

—Occupational training setting
—Self-contained special class in Special Education Center
—Self-contained special class in non-center
—Self-contained private facility
—Public residential school facility
—Private residential school facility
—Hospital
—Homebound program

— How many hours per week will the child spend with non-handi-capped students, and where will this time be spent? (Include recess, assemblies, lunch, other non-classroom activities.)
— Does the recommended program add up to 5½ hours a day of instructional time? (Not lunch, unless teaching the child to eat; not transportation.)
— Are there specific suggestions offered for what will be taught to your child? (Example: shapes, reading so many words, how to snap, toileting skills, etc.)
— Are these suggestions things that your child can already do at home? (If yes, be sure to tell the people at the conference.)
— Are there time limits on when your child will learn these things? Are these time limits realistic?
— Are there materials listed which will be used to teach your child the above things?
— Are there suggestions given for how you and the teacher will know when your child is able to do these things? (Example: four out of five times he/she will be able to tie shoes without assistance.)
— Are there suggestions given for how you can help the child at home?
— How often will there be contact between the home and the school, and what will be the nature of this contact? (Daily notes from the teacher, weekly newsletter to the entire class, etc.)

Reprinted with permission of The Association for Retarded Citizens, Philadelphia Chapter and The Bridge Vol. 1 No. 1, September 1981.

Who Decides If the Child Is
Ready for a Regular School?

If you understand the IEP process, you will see there is a "team approach" to determining objectives for education of the handicapped child. Of utmost importance is the fact that you, as a parent, are a part of the team that finalizes the IEP.

If your child has met all of the educational objectives there may be agreement that the child would do well in a regular school setting. Because the IEP must be reviewed annually, the question of placement in a different educational setting can be discussed. The important point to remember is that the educational needs of the child must be served. If the team feels this can be done in a regular school setting and you agree with the findings, plans may be made accordingly.

Placing a child with a handicap in a regular school setting is a major move and all of the ramifications of the change must be considered. Don't be afraid to ask questions!

If a Child Starts School After the Beginning of the
School Year, How Soon Should an IEP Be Developed?

Once a determination has been made that the child should be in a special education program, an IEP must be developed within 30 calendar days.

What If a Parent Cannot Attend an
IEP Meeting During School Hours?

The law and regulations governing the development of the IEP requires that the IEP meeting be held at times and places mutually convenient to parents and educators. It is therefore possible and often very likely that a meeting can be scheduled after school hours. Remember, the term is *mutually convenient.* Every effort should be made to work out a schedule with the teachers and administrators of the special education program in which your child is involved.

Must an IEP Be Developed for All Handicapped Children?

No. IEPs must be developed only for handicapped children requiring special education. Included in this group of children are only those falling under the definition of handicapping conditions given in Public Law 94-142. Some disabilities in no way affect a child's ability to function in regular classrooms and extracurricular activities.

Does the IEP Have to Be Written in Detail?

This question is not addressed in either the law or its regulations. Representatives of the U.S. Bureau of Education for the Handicapped have repeatedly stressed that the IEP is not meant to be a long, complicated form. Items included in the IEP should be concisely written.

The IEP is required to list only:

1. The child's present level of educational performance
2. Annual goals and short-term instructional objectives
3. Special education and related services to be provided
4. The extent of participation in regular education programs
5. Projected dates for initiation and expected duration of special services
6. Objective criteria and evaluation procedures to determine whether objectives are being met.

Can the IEP Be Developed Without the Presence of the Parents of the Handicapped Child in Question?

Yes, the IEP meeting can be held without the participation of parents if every effort was made by school personnel to involve the parents. There should be detailed documentation that the parents were notified of all rights and of the meeting in ample time before the actual date. Telephone calls and visits to the parent's home or workplace should be noted as being unproductive.

What Services Can I Seek for My Child Through the IEP?

The IEP meeting is usually attended by representatives of the school system (a school psychologist, the teacher, possibly a physician) and the parents of the potential student. The educational program and services that the child may need in order to reach present educational objectives are established.

The services, in addition to classroom instruction, may include physical education, physical therapy, occupational therapy, speech therapy, special instruction for the visually handicapped, psychological counseling, and various corrective and supportive services.

As a parent of a child with cerebral palsy or any other handicapping condition, you should be aware of the rules and regulations relating to the IEP. In that way, you will be able to obtain the many services your child may require.

How Can I Obtain More Information About the Purposes of the IEP?

The first step would be to talk with your child's teacher and the school principal. You would do well to come prepared for such a discussion by being familiar with the special education process.

To better understand the overall concept and purposes of Public Law 94-142, the Education for All Handicapped Children Act, contact your State Department of Education, Bureau of Special Education. They should have material on the Act that would describe your rights.

In addition, check with your local library to determine if the library carries any of the new publications referring to education of handicapped children. Two such publications are:

An Education Handbook for Parents of Handicapped Children by Stanley I. Mopsik and Judith A. Agard. Abt Books, Publishers, Cambridge, Mass. (cost $20)

The Compliance Manual, A Guide to the Rules and Regulations of the Education for All Handicapped Children Act, P.L. 94-142 by James C. Chalfant and Margaret Van Dusen Pysh. Pem Press, New Rochelle, N.Y. 10802 (cost $9.95)

Can School Districts Hire Physical Therapists?

Yes, according to Public Law 94-142, physical therapy is specifically mentioned as a "related service" that may be required to assist a handicapped child to benefit from special education and be included in the early identification and assessment of handicapping conditions in children.

Although it is not mandated that a physical therapist must be employed by a school district, the physical therapist is in a position to be of great help to school personnel and therapists are being hired in various school districts as full-time personnel or under special contract arrangements.

In addition to serving as advisors, physical therapists may be involved in developing the IEP by carrying out some of the recommendations made by the Committee on the Handicapped.

Physical therapists may give direct treatment services, act in a consulting role, work with school personnel in special activities periods, position children for maximum benefit in learning situations and conduct inservice programs on ambulation, transferring from wheelchairs to school chairs, and other activities of daily living.

Other professional personnel such as occupational therapists and speech therapists are also covered under Public Law 94-142 in the same manner described above.

What If My Child with Cerebral Palsy Does Not Meet All the Objectives of the IEP?

Because the IEP is not a legally binding contract, school teachers and districts cannot be held liable if the student does not reach certain objectives or does not make appropriate progress.

It is understood with the establishment of the IEP, however, that the school personnel will make every effort in working with the handicapped child to meet the special goals described in the IEP.

Must the Required Annual Review of the IEP Take Place on the Anniversary of the Original Planning Meeting?

No, although this is one possibility. The timing of these meetings is left to the discretion of the school system, but they must be scheduled sometime within a year of the last IEP meeting.

Should My Child's Teacher Be the Person Responsible for Letting Me Know About the IEP Meeting?

The school system is responsible for seeing that parents are notified of these meetings, in their native language if necessary.

Schools may designate this responsibility to anyone and, in many cases, it has been assigned to teachers. It should be noted that contacting parents for the IEP meeting may also be seen as an administrative responsibility which would leave the teachers more time to teach.

Are Teachers Required to Attend IEP Meetings After School Hours?

This possibility does exist. IEP planning meetings must be held at times and locations mutually convenient to parents and educators. They, therefore, in some instances could be held in a location other than the school and outside of the regular school hours (Rauth, 1981).

IEP planning meetings could conceivably be held during the summer.

Do Parents Have the Right to an Independent Educational Evaluation of Their Handicapped Child?

Yes. Each public agency must provide to parents, upon request, information on where an independent educational evaluation may be obtained. The parent has the right to such an evaluation at public expense whenever the parent disagrees with the evaluation obtained by the public agency.

The public agency must either pay for the independent evaluation or see that it is provided at no cost to the parent.

Is There Any Case in Which a Parent Would Be Denied an Independent Evaluation at Public Expense?

Yes. If the public agency initiated a due process hearing on its evaluation which was then shown to be appropriate, the parent would still have the right to an independent evaluation, but not at public expense.

Can Parent-Initiated Evaluations at Parent's Own Expense Be Considered in Determining the Child's Educational Program?

Yes. If a parent obtains an independent educational evaluation at private expense, it must be considered by the public agency in any decision made regarding provision of a free appropriate public education to the child or may be used as evidence at a due process hearing.

Evaluation criteria, however, must meet the state education agency's standards.

May Parents Inspect and Review All Education Records of Their Child?

Yes. Parents may inspect and review all education records with respect to identification, evaluation, and placement of the child and the provision of a free appropriate public education.

When Is Parental Consent Absolutely Required?

Parental consent is mandatory only before conducting a preplacement evaluation or initial placement of a handicapped child in a program providing special education and related services. Many implementors are not aware that any changes in a child's special education program after the initial placement are not subject to parental consent, although requirements of the individualized education program and prior notice must be met.

Parents may present complaints or grievances through the due process procedure at any time. Information on how this can be done will be made available to parents through the school district administrative personnel.

What Happens If Parents Refuse to Give Their Consent When Required?

State procedures govern the public agency in overriding a parent's refusal to consent in those states in which such consent is required by state law. Where there is no state law requiring consent before a handicapped child is evaluated or initially provided special education and related services, the agency may use due process hearing procedures established in Public Law 94-142. If the hearing or review officer upholds the agency, the agency may proceed without parental consent.

Once Parental Consent Has Been Given, Can It Be Revoked?

Yes. Parental consent is voluntary and may be revoked at any time.

Can the Public Agency Use Private Facilities for the Educational Needs of a Special Child?

Yes. States must see that eligible students receive a free appropriate public education. This is done through public agencies or institutions where appropriate services are available.

In cases in which such services are not available, a child may be placed, at public expense, in a private agency or institution that can meet the child's special needs. The state and/or local education agencies retain responsibility for assuring that these children's rights are protected under Public Law 94-142.

PROBLEMS IN AND OUT OF SCHOOL

Will My Child Always Be at the School in the Cerebral Palsy Center?

You may hear the term *less restrictive environment placements.* Through the concept of such placements, children with cerebral palsy may go into a regular school situation after being in a special program at a cerebral palsy center.

Under Public Law 94-142, each public agency must insure that handicapped children are educated with non-handicapped children to the maximum extent possible and that placement of a handicapped child outside the regular classroom occurs only when the nature or severity of the handicap is such that education in regular classes with the use of supplementary aids and services cannot be achieved satisfactorily.

The fundamental question is often how best to meet the handicapped child's needs. Because every child with cerebral palsy is different, parents should not consider placement of their child in a regular school as being automatic at a certain age. For the appropriate child, it should be the goal.

Can a Child with Cerebral Palsy Be Suspended from School for "Acting Up"?

Generally, a parent will find that a handicapped student may not be suspended for behavior that is typical of the particular handicapping condition. Suspension may be considered for such reasons as insubordination or disorderly conduct with the same rules applying to handicapped and nonhandicapped students.

If the question of suspension does arise because of the child's behavior, the assigned Committee of the Handicapped concerned with the child should be contacted.

Parents may also want to check with the Office of Children with Handicapping Conditions in their State Education Department for information on the rules applicable to suspension.

Must Alternative Instruction Be Provided to a Handicapped Student Who Has Been Formally Suspended from an Educational Program?

The answer to this question may vary in different states depending upon the Education Department's rules and regulations.

For example, in New York State, if a handicapped student has been suspended for 5 days (informal) or in excess of 5 days (formal), and the student is of compulsory attendance age, immediate steps should be taken for the attendance of the student or instruction offered elsewhere. This means that school districts should act reasonably promptly with due regard for the nature and circumstances of the particular case.

Furthermore, in such a situation, if the suspension is for more than 5 days, the Board of Education must provide the pupil or a person in parental relation an opportunity for a formal hearing. This involves the superintendent or Board of Education in conducting a formal hearing; and both should attempt to come to agreement as to the appropriate course of action to be taken in meeting the educational needs of the handicapped child.

(*Note:* This very question was written up in a newsletter issued by the State Education Department, New York, May 1981. Although circumstances for suspension may remain the same, parents should make every attempt to be familiar with the Education Department's rules and regulations in their own state.)

What Is the Difference Between Mainstreaming and Less Restrictive Environment Placements?

Sometimes the two terms are used synonymously; other times *mainstreaming* is used to mean placement of disabled students in regular classrooms.

Because in some cases, school systems rushed to mainstream as many disabled children as possible into regular classrooms, thereby hoping to save a considerable amount of money normally spent on special education, main-streaming developed a negative connotation. This type of placement obviously was not based on the individual needs of the child.

In federal legislation, *less restrictive environment place-ments* finally replaced mainstreaming as an attempt to over-come its tarnished image and better convey the continuum of alternative placements.

What Should the Lay and Professional Educator Know About the Handling of a Child with Cerebral Palsy?

With the growth of special programs for children with physical and mental handicaps, and the possibility of more of the children entering regular classes, teachers have an obligation to become more familiar with cerebral palsy and other conditions. In particular, they should be aware of the causes of cerebral palsy, the major classifications and characteristics related to the emotional, educational, and psychological growth, treatment approaches, the "team concept" in the management of the child, and community support services. Much of this information is made available through inservice education and graduate courses in the community.

The local cerebral palsy treatment facility or associa-tion can be asked to cooperate with people in special educa-tion and to work cooperatively in the best interests of children with cerebral palsy. Many professionals involved in habilitation of children with cerebral palsy are also available to work with teachers.

Of particular importance to the teacher in special education is a thorough understanding of Public Law 94-142.

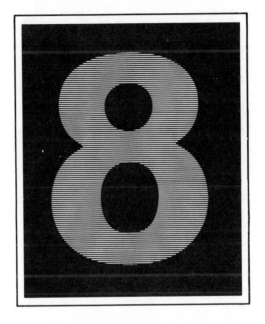

LIFE EXPERIENCES

How Can a Parent Obtain
Information on Governmental Services?

According to a publication from the Office of Information and Resources for the Handicapped, Washington, D.C. (1981), there is a national network of Federal Information Centers (FIC) available to guide citizens through the maze of agencies, programs and departments in the government to obtain the information they need. Centers are located in 41 key cities throughout the country. Residents in 43 other cities have direct access to their nearest FIC via local telephone tielines.

Questions concerning veteran's benefits, taxes, social security, regulations, and programs for disabled children are some of the routine subjects on which questions are fielded by the FIC staff. It has been reported that over 7.6 million people in 1980 dialed their local FIC for assistance. Staff specialists in many cities speak additional languages; Spanish is the most frequent second language.

There are statewide toll-free 800 numbers in Florida, Iowa, Kansas, Missouri, and Nebraska. Check your phone directory under Federal Information Centers, United States Government. A listing of all addresses and phone numbers is available from the:

> General Service Administration
> Federal Information Center
> Washington, DC 20405

FINANCIAL ASSISTANCE

Is There a Guide to Financial Assistance Available?

A compact guide is available through the Office of Information and Resources for the Handicapped, Department of Health and Human Services, Washington, D.C. 20201.

The publication is called, *Pocket Guide to Federal Help for the Disabled Person.* It describes the principal services applicable to individuals with developmental disabilities.

It is important to recognize that state and localities may provide additional services using their own resources. Check with your local, county, or state information office of the Department of Health or the Department of Social Services.

How About Receiving Medicaid?

Medicaid is a joint federal/state program to provide physical and related health care services to persons of low income.

Disabled persons, such as those with cerebral palsy, may be eligible for Medicaid on the basis of their income. Because eligibility is determined by each state program of public assistance on the basis of broad Federal guidelines, there are geographical differences between eligibility requirements and the types of services covered.

Generally, persons are eligible for Medicaid if they are receiving welfare or other public assistance benefits, Supplemental Security Income (SSI), or are blind or disabled.

The best way to obtain information about Medicaid services is to check with your local or state welfare or public assistance office. You may also want to write for information to:

Health Care Financing Administration—Medicaid
Room 4094   Switzer Building
330 Independence Avenue, S.W.
Washington, DC 20210

Can Adults with Cerebral Palsy Obtain Medicare?

Medicare services are available to persons over the age of 65 or to a disabled person who is entitled to social security disability benefits or railroad disability annuities for 2 consecutive years or more.

A disabled person will get hospital insurance automatically.

Specific problems and questions should be directed to your local social security office. It would be listed in the phone book under *United States Government.*

It is advisable to discuss benefits with a professional person, such as the social worker, at the treatment facility in your area. Do not wait until you actually need the services. Become familiar with the benefit program in advance.

What Are the Social Security Benefits for a Person with Cerebral Palsy?

There are two types of Social Security Disability Insurance benefits that are available:

1. Benefits for persons disabled since childhood, available if parents have paid into Social Security during their work lives.
2. Benefits for persons disabled as an adult, available through their own personal Social Security contributions when they were in the work force. This type generally does not involve the person with cerebral palsy because the condition usually is present from childhood.

Monthly benefits may be paid to persons disabled before age 22 who continue to be disabled, and whose parent (or grandparent under certain circumstances) receives social security retirement or disability benefits or whose insured parent dies.

Persons who are disabled and whose income and resources are very limited may be eligible to receive Supplemental Security Income (SSI) benefits. SSI is designed to provide minimum income for those persons whose disability prevents them from gainful employment and who may not have been able to contribute to the regular Social Security system.

Financial eligibility for SSI is very complex. You may have some income and still be eligible for benefits. SSI may also be available to disabled children if a person is under 18 years of age, not married, and not the head of a household. That person is considered a child under SSI guidelines.

Information on benefits may be obtained through your local Social Security office or through the social services department of the treatment facility with which you are best acquainted.

RESIDENTIAL CARE—RESPITE SERVICES

Are Parents of Children with Cerebral Palsy Always Considered Guardians?

If a child is 18 years old or older, the parent is not automatically considered a guardian. The parent must have legal authorization by an official proceeding in the Surrogates Court.

Parents of mentally retarded or emotionally handicapped children have no legal control or supervision, financial or otherwise, after the child reaches 18 years of age.

According to the Legal and Governmental Relations Committee of a major cerebral palsy center, legal guardianship can be established before the child reaches age 18 if the parents believe the child will require some lifetime guidance or supervision.

Guardianship is usually divided into two parts—guardian of the person and guardian of the property. One person can be named to handle both.

It is important for parents of severely handicapped children to give the concept of guardianship attention, for as the child grows older, thought must be given to the future when parents are not around to oversee the child's needs.

What Will Happen to Our Child When We Are Gone?

This is a matter of grave concern to all parents of children and adults with cerebral palsy.

Fortunately, many of the associations involved in programming for the handicapped have legal committees and trust officers to advise and discuss what plans should be made for the person with cerebral palsy in the event that parents are no longer alive.

Guardianship may be considered. Establishing a trust fund to care for the child after the parents are gone is another method of assuring continuity of care. At parent meetings, programs are often presented to explain how the child is made a recipient of funding through a will.

The fact that certain people are eligible for Medicaid is another possible source of support. This may tie in with the move to establish more small community facilities within areas served by a cerebral palsy association.

Concern for the child's future after the death of the parents has always been a major topic of discussion among the parents. With leaders of public and private agencies involved in planning, with state and federal funding and with the involvement of concerned parents, residential alternatives are becoming increasingly available. It is not likely that an individual with cerebral palsy will be left "out on the street."

Why Doesn't the State Provide More Acceptable Residential Schools for the Moderately to Severely Handicapped Child?

Since the mid-1970s, there has been a major trend to eliminate large residential centers and institutions primarily serving persons with retardation in what is known as the *deinstitutionalization process.* In addition, as community services have developed there are more resources available to most children with disabilities in their own community.

In spite of the generally accepted philosophy that it is better for the child with cerebral palsy to be at home in a family unit rather than in a residential setting, there are circumstances in which the child may have better opportunities for development in a residential facility. There has been extremely slow growth, however, in establishing special residential schools. Most states do not see maintaining disabled children in residential schools as their prime responsibility. Those facilities that are available are usually operated by voluntary agencies, by religious groups, or on a private basis. Residential programs are very costly to operate and need a large well-trained staff. Tuition may be out of the reach of the average parent. Eventually, a compromise may be necessary, wherein many options become available—from acceptable residential schools run by the state to community-based facilities having public and private funding.

What is "Respite Care"?

Parents of children with cerebral palsy often feel they cannot leave their child for any length of time, for fear that no one else will give them proper care. Many parents have described lives in which they have never had an evening out or a weekend away, because their major concern was meeting the needs of their child.

Respite care has been designed to allow trained individuals to give some relief time to parents.

Finding a suitable definition for *respite care* is difficult. The term respite care has been defined in many ways by care providers, with little general agreement on the question of what it consists of or what it is intended to accomplish (Warren and Dickman, 1981).

Generally, respite care is a service that offers temporary relief to the primary caregiver (usually the parents). Temporary relief could be provided for a period from an hour or two to several months. The service would allow parents to be relieved of the constant care of the child with cerebral palsy in nonemergency situations.

For emergency situations, parents should contact the medical facility with which they are most familiar. Arrangements for temporary care usually can be made through the social services department. It is advisable to be aware of what services are available in your community before the emergency need arises.

How Does a Parent Obtain Respite Services?

Respite care may include a variety of services such as in-home sitters, home-care workers, companions, and week-end and summer recreation programs. Within many parts of the country, a United Cerebral Palsy affiliate may be able to provide such services. If the UCP agency does not have the program, usually one of the professional staff will be aware of what resources can be made available to the parents.

For further information, there is a useful publication:

For This Respite, Much Thanks, by Rachel D. Warren and Irving R. Dickman, a combined philosophy and how-to-do-it manual for respite care development. This 144-page paperback is available for $3.00 from:

United Cerebral Palsy Associations, Inc.
66 East 34 St.
New York, NY 10016

VOCATIONAL TRAINING

What Vocational Training Is Available to Adults with Cerebral Palsy?

Under the direction of the state agency known as the Bureau or Department of Vocational Rehabilitation, there are several types of vocational services available to the individual with cerebral palsy.

Much of the training will depend upon the severity of the condition of the individual. However, severity should not preclude the possibility of accomplishing what a person with cerebral palsy wants to do.

Vocational training has been expanded into many communities through the efforts of voluntary agencies who operate evaluation and training centers with support from the state agency responsible for vocational rehabilitation.

Training may be available that would lead to placement in a sheltered workshop, a commercial firm, or a career field. The training received will depend upon the mental and physical abilities of the individual.

Are Job Opportunities Available for the Adult with Cerebral Palsy?

The adult with cerebral palsy will have competition for employment even though he or she may feel highly qualified.

Numerous examples of individuals with cerebral palsy can be described in which the talents and abilities of the disabled person are not recognized by potential employers. Much remains to be done to educate the general public and make employers aware of the abilities of the individual.

Those adults with cerebral palsy who do demonstrate their abilities may eventually find satisfaction and acceptance on the job. Many stories can be told of the years of frustration faced by adults with cerebral palsy before being accepted for employment. There is the occasional computer expert, the researcher, the psychologist, the film producer, the social worker, the engineer . . . but generally, finding a rewarding position will be difficult.

The adult with cerebral palsy should be prepared for an uphill battle. This becomes more obvious during difficult economic times and periods of large scale unemployment within the general population.

What Is the Availability of Sheltered Workshops?

It is estimated that there are as many as 2,000 sheltered workshops maintained by voluntary associations and nonprofit organizations in the United States.

Adults with cerebral palsy who have severe physical or mental disabilities are not conspicuously present in certain types of workshops in which speed and commercialism are emphasized. More often, the adult with severe cerebral palsy is in a workshop or training program sponsored by such agencies as the United Cerebral Palsy Association or those established primarily for persons with retardation.

How Can I Obtain a Listing of Sheltered Workshops?

The most complete listing of facilities described and classified as sheltered workshops is available from the:

Association of Rehabilitation Facilities
5530 Wisconsin Avenue, Suite 955
Washington, DC 20015

In What Fields Have Those Persons with Cerebral Palsy Succeeded?

A study of adults with cerebral palsy (Schleichkorn and Manus, 1971) described the many occupations in which the adults were involved. It would appear that the adult with cerebral palsy can succeed in almost any type of work provided they have the intellectual capacity. Among the fields listed in the study are:

Printer	Social Worker
County Surveyor	Custodial Supervisor
Statistician	Professor
Certified Public	Clerk
Accountant	Receptionist
Executive Secretary	Administrator
Artist	Attorney
Engineer	Store Owner
Insurance Executive	Janitor
Computer Programmer	Public Relations
Electrician	Librarian
Writer	Workshop Supervisor
Actuary	Banker
Teacher	Secretary
Bookkeeper	Economist
Research Assistant	
Nurseryman	

There are adults with cerebral palsy who have gone into such professional fields as psychology, speech therapy, physical therapy, rehabilitation counseling, social services, education, recreation, and medicine.

Parents should be aware of early exposure to responsibility, to opportunities for interpersonal skills to develop, to hobbies that may lead to increased attention span and interests, to prevocational interest evaluations, and to prevocational skills such as travel and budgeting.

Are There Advantages to Employers Hiring the Handicapped?

Probably the most important benefit to an employer who hires handicapped people is the knowledge that the company will have productive members who have demonstrated outstanding safety habits and minimal absenteeism.

It should be noted that the Rehabilitation Act of 1973 recognizes that not every disabled applicant for a position may be qualified to perform every available task. A handicapped person can be employed to do a specific task requiring reasonable accommodations to perform that job effectively.

Employer studies indicate that disabled workers are capable of holding their own and do not increase workers' compensation costs.

An adult with cerebral palsy may want to take this type of information to an employer when seeking a position.

What Are the Federal Requirements for Hiring the Handicapped?

The Rehabilitation Act of 1973 was designed to improve employment opportunities for disabled people. The Act requires employers with more than $2,500 in federal contracts or subcontracts to take affirmative action in the hiring and promotion of those people considered to be disabled.

The law further requires employers receiving grants and other federal financial assistance to be nondiscriminatory in considering disabled people for employment.

The requirements of the Rehabilitation Act affect about 3 million or one-half of the nation's employers.

What Recourse Does a Person with Cerebral Palsy Have in the Event of Discrimination in Seeking Employment?

If the employer's business is involved with a Federal Government contract for more than $2,500, any person with a handicap who suffers discrimination may submit a signed complaint with the Office of Federal Contract Compliance of the Department of Labor, Washington, D.C.

Further information is included in a special publication, *Affirmative Action to Employ Handicapped People.* It is a pocket guide to the regulations of the affirmative action section requirements of Section 503 of the Rehabilitation Act of 1973.

Write the President's Committee on Employment of the Handicapped, Washington, D.C. 20210. The pamphlet is available at no charge.

SPECIAL EQUIPMENT

Where Can I Get Information on Clothes for Disabled People?

A special publication, *Clothing for Handicapped People,* has been prepared and published at the University of Arizona for the President's Committee on Employment of the Handicapped.

The publication concentrates on acquiring or adapting clothes that fit and allow handicapped persons to easily dress themselves. The information is intended to inform the public of what has been developed and accomplished in the field of clothing for people with special needs. It includes sources of information on clothing and shoes for people with specific handicapping conditions.

Available from:

> The President's Committee on Employment
> of the Handicapped
> 1111 20th St. N.W.
> Washington, DC 20036

Are There Books on How to Make Special Clothing for Disabled People?

There are a variety of publications that offer information and designs on special clothing for the disabled.

Write directly to the sources listed below or check with your local library or treatment center to determine if the information is available locally.

Self-Help Clothing by E. B. Hotte. Available for $1.50 (plus 75¢ postage) from:

> National Easter Seal Society
> 2023 West Ogden Ave.
> Chicago, IL 60612

Clothing for the Handicapped, Aged and Other People with Special Needs by A. M. Hoffman. Available for $12.50 from:

> Charles C Thomas, Publisher
> Springfield, IL

Clothing Designs for the Handicapped by A. Kernaleguen. Available for $15 from:

> University of Alberta Press
> Edmonton, Alberta
> Canada

Clothes to Fit Your Needs for the Physically Limited by J. Yep. Available from the:

> Connecticut Cooperative Extension Service
> 322 N. Main St.
> Wallingford, CT 06492

Clothing for the Handicapped. Available from:
Sister Kenny Institute
2727 Chicago Ave.
Minneapolis, MN 55407

LeChic. Offers suggestions for clothing adaptations upon request. Write to:
LeChic
P.O. Box 22552
Sacramento, CA 95882

Adapt Your Own. Available from:
Office of Independent Study
Division of Continuing Education
P.O. Box 2167
University, AL 34586

Can Special Clothes for the Disabled Be Purchased?

There are several manufacturers and organizations that offer special clothing or adaptations for the disabled, including persons confined to wheelchairs. Information and catalogs may be obtained by writing directly to the company.

Disabled Clothiers of California
6950 21st Ave.
Sacramento, CA 95820

Fashion Able, Catalog of Adaptive Clothing
Rocky Hill, NJ 08553

Fashions Handee for You
7674 Park Ave.
Lowville, NY 13367
(Catalog $1, returnable with first order)

Vocational Guidance and Rehabilitation Service
Clothing Aids
2239 East 55 St.
Cleveland, OH
($1.00)

P.T.L. Designs, Inc.
P.O. Box 364
Stillwater, OK 74074
($1.00)

The Natural Creations, Textile Research Center
Texas Tech University
Lubbock, TX 79409

Men's Fashions for the Wheelchair Set
Wm. F. Leineweber, Inc.
Brunswick Building, 69 W. Washington
Chicago, IL 60602

Levis: Custom jeans for people with special needs
Levis, E.P.P. Dept. 8888
6621 Geyser Springs Rd.
Little Rock, AK 77209

On the Rise (formerly I Can Do It Myself)
Clothing for special people with special needs
2282 Four Oaks Grange Road
Eugene, OR 97405
(Catalog available, $1.00)

What Is "Normalization"?

Many publications dealing with persons with developmental disabilities often refer to the term *normalization.*

Based upon a concept first promoted in Sweden in 1969 by Bengt Nirje, normalization then referred to providing persons with mental retardation experiences and lifestyles that are usually experienced by nonhandicapped individuals. Nirje explains normalization as a "means of making available to the mentally retarded patterns and conditions of everyday life which are as close as possible to the norms and patterns of the mainstream of society."

Normalization may also refer to any group of "devalued" people. A major proponent of the normalization concept, Dr. Wolf Wolfensberger, offers one definition as "the use of culturally valued means in order to enable people to live culturally valued lives."

SEX EDUCATION AND MARRIAGE

How Do You Explain the "Facts of Life" to a Young Person with Cerebral Palsy?

When the subject comes up, parents will realize how normal their child may be. Questions should be discussed and answered frankly to the extent of the understanding displayed by the individual with cerebral palsy. Care should be taken not to overwhelm the child with too many pieces of information at one time.

Specific materials have been published on sex education which will prove helpful to parents. Generally, materials prepared for children who are not disabled would be applicable.

Parents who are uncomfortable with the subject should look into what services may be available from community agencies serving the handicapped or to religious affiliations. Parent "rap" groups may be another source of support.

There are various sources for publications that could be of great help to parents. (see the next question)

Have Special Materials Been Prepared Dealing with Sex Information for People with Cerebral Palsy?

Studies have been done on sexual activities for the disabled and special materials have been published to assist parents in guiding the sexual education of their handicapped child. Such material is applicable to those with cerebral palsy.

For a listing of books and pamphlets on sex education write:

Ed-U Press
P.O. Box 583
Fayetteville, NY 13066

Another important source for special publications is

SIECUS (Sex Information and Education
Council of the United States)
84 Fifth Ave.
New York, NY 10011

A 43-page bibliography on *Sex Education for Individuals with Developmental Disabilities* is available through the University of Iowa. This material lists works specifically for and about the developmentally disabled and contains general sex education information as well. Publishers are included in the listing. Send $3.75 to:

> Campus Store, Room 30
> Iowa Memorial Union, University of Iowa
> Iowa City, IA 52242

Can Adults with Cerebral Palsy Marry?

As social groups serving people with handicaps develop within many communities, you can expect more adults with cerebral palsy to have opportunities to meet and foster friendships that could lead to marriage. This should not come as a surprise to parents. Because adults with cerebral palsy have the same sexual drives and emotional feelings as other people do, marriages will be considered.

Laws do not prevent marriages between handicapped people. . .only families do. Much depends upon the attitude of the parents, friends, and relatives. With appropriate thought, planning, and consideration of the many factors involved in making a success of marriage, it is likely that the matrimonial ceremony will take place.

Examples of couples with cerebral palsy who have been married may be found in many communities. Many are likely to be known to the local United Cerebral Palsy Association.

Of particular interest to parents concerned with marriage and their disabled offspring is a 12 page booklet, *Sexual Rights for the People. . . Who Happen to be Handicapped* by Sol Gordon. Available for $1 (plus minimum shipping charge of $1) from the:

> Human Policy Press
> P.O. Box 127
> Syracuse, NY 13210

Do Adults with Cerebral Palsy Tend to Marry Other Handicapped People?

There are many verified situations in which adults with cerebral palsy marry each other and manage quite well as independent community citizens.

In 1965, a major study of 586 persons with cerebral palsy was conducted in Israel (Margulec, 1966). Among the group studied were 21 persons who were married and one widow. According to the study report, of these, 9 persons were mildly disabled, 11 were moderately so, and 2 were severely disabled. Eleven cases had healthy spouses and 11 had disabled spouses. Among the disabilities in addition to cerebral palsy were blindness, post-polio, mental retardation, and muscular dystrophy.

The adult with cerebral palsy who has many opportunities to socialize with nondisabled people may find a "normal" mate. This is more likely to occur with the mildly affected person with cerebral palsy who may not need the services of an organization to plan recreational activities.

The mildly involved adult with cerebral palsy who goes to college and is able to obtain employment may have just as many opportunities to meet a member of the opposite sex as does anyone else.

The individual with cerebral palsy who is limited physically and depends upon an agency for the handicapped to plan all the recreational and social programs is often stymied in the desire to step out of the world of the disabled. This certainly limits the opportunity to meet anyone other than disabled people.

It is the capacity for shared interests and shared responsibilities, however, which makes or breaks any marriage, not the disability of either or both partners.

Are Normal Sex Relations Possible Between Couples with Cerebral Palsy?

Normal?. . .the range of physical limitations accompanying the condition of cerebral palsy often may eliminate the word *normal.* Much of the sexual activities of the couple will depend on their physical abilities.

Publications available at any bookstore are quite explicit on sex acts (including illustrations). Adults with cerebral palsy have indicated sexual fulfillment is possible with experience and experimentation. It is helpful for the adults to participate in social groups as programming often includes sex education.

Referring specifically to participation in sexual activities, one couple interviewed stated, "We find a way."

How Can a Couple with Cerebral Palsy Manage a Baby?

There may be difficulty in being able to handle certain aspects of baby care by a handicapped mother. It would be to the advantage of the family to obtain some special training before the baby arrives. Imagine trying to diaper an active infant if the mother has many involuntary movements (athetosis). You can be sure it is not impossible, however, and the mother will find a way.

There are many examples of parents with cerebral palsy successfully raising families. Bringing a baby into the home may require some extra assistance and support from other family members or from personnel in community agencies. A local voluntary agency or social service group may have just the kind of help required. The parents should not wait until the child arrives to make special arrangements. This should be done well in advance.

If an occupational therapist is available for consultation, make the contact. OTs are exceptionally well-qualified to offer suggestions, adaptations, or innovations that would make the activities of daily life easier for the entire family.

Can a Woman with Cerebral Palsy Have a Normal Pregnancy If She Has a Tendency to Fall Often?

Every attempt should be made to prevent the expectant mother from falling. This could be done by using an appliance such as a cane, walker, or crutch. Seek the opinion of professional personnel at a cerebral palsy center or other treatment facility. Although the mother-to-be may consider use of an appliance to be cumbersome, greater consideration should be given to maintaining the normal development of the pregnancy and protection of the fetus. In that way, the pregnancy could be uncomplicated.

How Does a Woman with Cerebral Palsy Manage a Pregnancy?

The pregnancy should be managed the same as with any other female. Appropriate prenatal care is most important. The difference that cerebral palsy may make should be of concern to the physician caring for the mother-to-be. The physician should be aware of the possibility of any and all risks and what precautions may be necessary to bring about a normal delivery. This is especially important for the female who has spastic adductor muscles that cause a scissor-like gait.

Planning for the delivery takes on an important meaning for the couple with cerebral palsy, perhaps more so than for a nondisabled couple. Both partners should not hesitate to discuss any aspects of the pregnancy with the physician.

What Is the Best Birth Control Method for Persons with Cerebral Palsy If They Get Married and Do Not Want to Have Children?

Without getting into any moral or religious issues, if the couple is sure they do not want children, sterilization of the female or a vasectomy for the male may be considered. This should be carefully thought out and discussed with a physician openly and frankly.

Actually, the same methods of birth control available to the nondisabled population are available to those with cerebral palsy.

Adults with cerebral palsy will find Planned Parenthood services have personnel knowledgeable and specially trained to meet the needs of the disabled population.

Specific information may also be obtained from the:

Coalition on Sexuality and Disability
122 East 23 Street
New York, NY 10010

LIFE EXPECTANCY

Is Life Expectancy
Shortened By Having Cerebral Palsy?

Most of the research on life expectancy and cerebral palsy was done before 1960. Various studies indicated that the mortality rate for children with cerebral palsy was higher than that of the general population.

In one of the primary texts on cerebral palsy, Crothers and Paine (1959) wrote: "It is clear that the majority of the cerebral palsied have a considerable life expectancy, and that those who do not reach adult life most commonly die between the ages of 5 and 20 years."

Another major study described a follow-up of 3,108 persons with cerebral palsy and included mortality rates. The report by Schlesinger, Allaway, and Petlin (1959) found the death rate of 9.6 per 10,000 person-years among males was 13 times the expected rate. Among females, the rate was 8.5 per 1,000 person-years, or 17 times the expected rate. The report also indicated that those persons with cerebral palsy who had severe physical limitations had a mortality rate 27 to 30 times greater than expected in the corresponding age-sex groups of the general population. Those persons with cerebral palsy with mild physical involvement had a mortality rate from 4 to 5 times greater than expected.

Of special interest in the Schlesinger study were the findings related to the very severely involved persons with mental retardation who were in state institutions. This group had a mortality rate about 30 times greater than expected based on accepted mortality rates in the general population.

Today there are many influences that could change the old statistics. With early recognition of neurological impairment, the saving of premature infants, various antibiotics, and the availability of health care services, it becomes obvious that new long-term studies on mortality and cerebral palsy are needed.

Can a Person with Cerebral Palsy Obtain Life Insurance?

Various companies have different policies regarding insurance for anyone with a disability. For persons who have cerebral palsy, usually, each case is underwritten on an individual basis. Most companies are willing to consider applicants who have special problems, but such firms may have some specific riders attached to the policy.

A new program of life insurance designed especially for individuals with cerebral palsy is offered by Unity Mutual Life Insurance Company with the endorsement of the United Cerebral Palsy Associations, Inc. Unity Life has developed special underwriting guidelines expressly for this program. Although the condition of cerebral palsy alone will not automatically exclude an applicant from being issued a standard life insurance policy, Unity Life makes no guarantee that a standard life insurance policy will be issued. For further information contact:

> Underwriting Department
> Unity Mutual Life Insurance Company
> One Unity Plaza
> Syracuse, NY 13215

HIGHER EDUCATION

Should an Adult with Cerebral Palsy Seek Admission to College?

If the individual with cerebral palsy is capable of handling the academic work, qualifies for admission, and is desirous of obtaining a college education, there is no reason to deny such a person the experience of going to college.

Many adults with cerebral palsy who seek a secure position in employment feel that a college education is necessary. Despite physical limitations, there are outstanding examples of individuals with cerebral palsy who manage to handle their difficulties and obtain a college degree.

Not every university or college campus may be architecturally barrier free and this may pose problems in getting around the campus. The old adage, "where there's a will, there's a way" seems to be the theme for many handicapped people on college campuses.

Parents who are concerned about their handicapped son or daughter going off on their own to a campus may want to seek out an individual with cerebral palsy who was successful in meeting the challenge. Such persons can usually be contacted through the local United Cerebral Palsy organization. Some parents may be surprised to hear the college-educated adult does not think the education offered security in employment. The adult with cerebral palsy who intends to go for a higher education must be strongly motivated. The most important aspect of seeking a college education should relate to the individual's career goal or objective. Good vocational and career guidance is vital!

Are There Any Federal Grants or Tuition Assistance for Persons with Cerebral Palsy Interested in Higher Education?

Tuition assistance for qualified disabled persons is available from the state vocational rehabilitation agency. A person with cerebral palsy who has the intellectual ability to participate in a higher education program probably will be recognized while still in high school. Through the involvement of the vocational rehabilitation agency, a wide variety of services can be made available. These include funding for special programs, transportation, tuition assistance, and special equipment. Although the grants do not come directly from the federal agency to the student, the program is made available in every state to persons with disabilities. Check with the federal office at the following address for specific information about the state programs:

Office of Handicapped Individuals
Office of Human Development
U.S. Department of Health and Human Services
200 Independence Ave., S.W.
Washington, DC 20201

What Colleges Are Best Suited for an Adult with Cerebral Palsy?

Some 500 colleges have eliminated architectural barriers to accommodate disabled students. Many have special offices and personnel to ease the transition for the disabled student into the higher education environment. There are two major publications you should check out. Your local library may be a good starting point. The publications are:

The College Guide for Students With Disabilities by Elinor Gollay and Alwina Bennet. Available from:
Abt Books
55 Wheeler Street
Cambridge, MA 02138

Getting Through College With a Disability: A Summary of Services Available on 500 Campuses for Students With Handicapping Conditions. Available from:
The President's Committee on Employment
of the Handicapped
Washington, DC 20210

What Allowances Will a College Make for a Student with Cerebral Palsy?

The Rehabilitation Act of 1973, Section 504, prohibits discrimination against students who are disabled when attending an educational facility which receives federal aid. The regulations that implement Section 504 place certain responsibilities upon the facility so that the needs of the disabled persons will be met. Therefore, if a student with cerebral palsy enters a particular college or university, he or she should be sure the regulations related to Section 504 are known to the facility. Most major institutions have a special office to meet the needs of the disabled. The student with cerebral palsy must make himself known to that office so that mandated support is made available. For example, the university must provide all students equal opportunity to participate in student activities; assure that campus buildings conform to the structural requirements set by federal law; provide nondiscriminatory standards in all academic areas and appropriate educational aids when necessary; provide housing comparable in cost, convenience, and accessibility to that provided to nondisabled students; make available total health care services and insurances; and provide nondiscriminatory financial aid programs, scholarships, student employment, counseling, academic advisement, career development, and job placement.

It is advisable to visit a campus before making the final decision to apply to the school and meet with a representative of the Office of the Disabled or the Equal Opportunity/ Affirmative Action Office. Many allowances are made for the disabled student because of Section 504 and it is important that the person with cerebral palsy be aware of the rules and regulations. Details can usually be obtained through the state vocational rehabilitation agency.

If Adults with Cerebral Palsy Have College Training, Do They Stand a Better Chance for Employment?

There is no guarantee that a college education completed by the adult with cerebral palsy will mean success in employment. This is true of any person. Much will depend on the goal orientation of the handicapped individual, placement, and the ability to do the job. There are many adults with cerebral palsy who, after obtaining a college education, have become frustrated with the lack of opportunity to put their training to work. One needs to be very realistic as to one's career goal.

Today, with antidiscrimination laws, one would assume that the college-educated adults with cerebral palsy would have no difficulty in being placed in a situation for which they have been trained. Ask some of these adults, and you will find some very disappointed people out in the real world.

MOBILITY

Why Don't All Public Buildings Have Easy Access for Wheelchairs?

Public Law 90-480, the Architectural Barriers Act of 1968, seeks to make any facility built or supported by federal funds barrier free. Much has been accomplished since the legislation was enacted. In some situations, the changes have been obvious, as in museums, libraries, state and federal buildings, and county centers. There still is a great need to call attention to those facilities that are not entirely accessible. If a private contractor is planning a facility without thought of accessibility, then all the campaigns to educate the public have failed. There must be constant awareness, pressure, and education to make all people realize that certain changes in architectural design will benefit everyone.

The U.S. Code, Title 42, Section 4151-56 states:

> Any building constructed or leased in whole or in part with federal funds must be made accessible to and usable by the physically handicapped.

This law applies to any building designed, constructed, or altered after standards of accessibility were developed by the General Services Administration, the Department of

Housing and Urban Development, and the Department of Defense.

Why Aren't All Voting Places Required to Be Accessible to the Handicapped?

More and more states now have legislation requiring voting sites to be completely accessible to the disabled. Check with your local Board of Elections for your area. You may also want information from the League of Women Voters. They offer listings of all state and local elected officials. If your voting sites are not accessible, let your legislators know that you want a change. This can be done as an individual or through your cerebral palsy association.

Can an Adult with Cerebral Palsy Learn to Drive?

Reasonably, one would have to consider the severity of the handicap and the intellectual ability of the individual. If the desire is there to learn to drive, and appropriate adaptations can be made to a vehicle, it certainly may be possible for the adult to drive. Once again, contact with a local agency serving the handicapped may give you an opportunity to gain first-hand knowledge about successful drivers who are handicapped.

The American Automobile Association offers a listing of training and evaluation facilities in a booklet, *The Handicapped Driver's Mobility Guide* (DeLellis, 1978). Check with any local AAA office.

How Does an Adult with Cerebral Palsy Obtain a License to Drive?

The mobility afforded to an adult with cerebral palsy through driving a car will lead to greater independence.

In completing the driver's license application, you usually find a question related to the individual's having a disability that requires special attention by the Department of Motor Vehicles. The procedure will require an evaluation by a department inspector to determine what car modifications will be necessary to operate the vehicle. For example, if you cannot use your legs for control of the vehicle, adapted hand controls may be in order. Once the required car modifications are installed and the handicapped driver feels proficient behind the wheel, he or she must take the required road test. It is the same test offered to everyone in the state. In New York State, it was reported that only 10% of all handicapped applicants fail their road test as compared to 40% of the nonhandicapped population. This probably is due to the special training required and the determination of the handicapped persons. Adults with cerebral palsy may not be able to rely on public transportation; therefore, they must depend on their own skills.

Can Someone Who Is Subject to Seizures Obtain a Driver's License?

You should check with the Department of Motor Vehicles to determine what special restrictions or regulations may be in effect in your state. It appears that in most areas an applicant for a driver's license with a history of seizures must answer "Yes" to a question pertaining to seizures and related disorders on the application. Then the application, together with a brief written history and recommendation from the applicant's personal physician, is sent to a Medical Review Board of the Department of Motor Vehicles. The board will review the history and either approve or disapprove the application. Although individual circumstances vary, the board generally requires the applicant to be seizure-free for a minimum period of 18 months, with or without seizure-control medication.

The adult with cerebral palsy and controlled seizures must consider all of the ramifications of driving, but, certainly, it is possible to obtain a license.

**Where Can an Adult with Cerebral
Palsy Obtain Special Information About
Adaptations Necessary to Drive a Car?**

There are several possibilities. Write for information to:

The Paralyzed Veterans of America, Inc.
4330 East-West Highway, Suite 300
Washington, DC 20014

or check with your library for a copy of *Serving Physically Disabled People. . . An Information Handbook for All Libraries* by Ruth Velleman (1979). The book includes a listing of some 29 manufacturers of automobile hand controls, assistive devices, and vehicle modifiers.

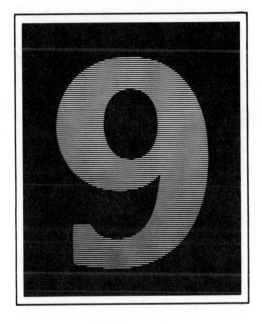

RESEARCH

What Can Research Do to Prevent Cerebral Palsy?

The aims of the United Cerebral Palsy Research and Educational Foundation include finding ways to prevent cerebral palsy as well as methods to improve the functioning of children and adults who have the condition. Much has been done in support of research, most notably in prevention of cerebral palsy. The Foundation has given grants that have contributed to several important scientific advances, such as: the rubella vaccine, which protects mothers from infection with German measles; a safe and effective light treatment for jaundice of the newborn; a method of identifying high-risk newborns; and development of the fetal heart monitor. The Foundation's Research Council has also pinpointed three major areas for study that involve prevention of cerebral palsy. One such area is prevention of prematurity; another involves the ability to manage prematurely born babies in neonatal intensive care units; and the third area deals with the control of infections that occur in the newborn during fetal development. Improvement of prenatal and infant care has also contributed to the reduction in cerebral palsy. Continued research in this area will hopefully see further advances in establishing total services for pregnant women.

Voluntary agencies such as UCP and the federal government working with professional personnel are striving for further reduction in the number of children born with cerebral palsy.

What Type of Research Is Being Done in Cerebral Palsy?

Governmental and private organizational funding is heavily directed to all types of research activities related directly and indirectly to prevent cerebral palsy and improve the functioning of those children and adults who have cerebral palsy. A major funding agency is the United Cerebral Palsy

Research and Educational Foundation. In 1980, Dr. Leon Sternfeld, UCP's Medical Director, reported that 34 research projects were currently underway under the Foundation's program (United Cerebral Palsy Associations, 1981). Among the areas being investigated are: prevention of prematurity; improved management of very low birthweight infants, including early detection; sources of damage to the fetus and newborn; study of commonly used medications that may affect the fetal nervous system; means of controlling spasticity; evaluation of chronic cerebellar stimulation; methods of analyzing mobility and gait as a means for improving orthopedic surgery; devices and methods of producing nonverbal communication; and the use of orthotics in increasing mobility. Federal research programs also have been geared toward better understanding of the neurological system, prevention and improving the lifestyle of the country's handicapped people. Another area of research in which the federal government is involved relates to making existing technology known, not only to scientists, researchers, and other professionals, but to the handicapped person as well.

Detailed reports on research projects may be obtained by writing to the Department of Health and Human Services, Washington, D.C., the United Cerebral Palsy Research and Educational Foundation, 66 East 34th Street, New York, N.Y. 10016, and/or the National Easter Seal Society, 2023 West Ogden Avenue, Chicago, Ill. 60612.

How Can Research Help My Child?

Many parents are concerned that present research has little effect on their child. This may be so when related to research toward prevention of cerebral palsy because the child already has the condition. One must still agree with the importance of trying to prevent other children from having cerebral palsy. Research has already demonstrated there can be a reduction in cerebral palsy, mental retardation, and other developmental disabilities.

Those parents who have other, nondisabled children would want to reduce the possibilities of any chance that their offspring would have to cope with a child with cerebral palsy in their family.

Research also involves more than the stereotypical sterile laboratory. Every treatment center, classroom, residential facility, or program is a site for research. Studies done on independent living, treatment techniques, educational activities, residential care, engineering, and biomechanics, all will allow today's children and adults with cerebral palsy to function better. Research is an ongoing process and must be encouraged and supported!

GLOSSARY OF TERMS

There are many terms commonly used by professional personnel that may not be explained to the parents of children with cerebral palsy or other disabilities.

The glossary is based on material originally prepared by members of the New York Chapter, American Physical Therapy Association Task Force Physical Therapists in School Settings, in 1979.

The information will be helpful to parents by offering an understanding of some of the terminology often used when professionals discuss their child's case.

Special acknowledgement is given to the Task Force, Virginia Browning, Chairman, for granting permission to use the material.

Abduction movement of a limb away from the body.

Adduction movement of a limb toward the body.

Agonist the muscle that is the prime mover in a specific movement.

Antagonist the muscle that is directly opposite in movement to the agonist.

ATNR (asymmetrical tonic neck reflex) performed by turning head of a child to one side slowly and holding it in position for 15 seconds. Response in newborn to 3 months: extension of chin arm with flexion of opposite arm or any increase in tone. After 5 months of age, the consistent response is abnormal.

Atrophy deterioration or loss of tissue, especially muscle tissue.

Bilateral pertaining to use of both sides of the body in a simultaneous and parallel fashion.

Body image complete awareness of one's body and its possibilities of movement and performance.

CCS chronic cerebellar stimulation.

Cerebral palsy   the result of damage to or maldevelopment of the brain, occurring *in utero* or in earliest childhood. The lesion is nonprogressive and acts on an immature brain, interfering with its normal process of maturation. The term *cerebral palsy* comprises a group of conditions of great variety. With respect to the motor handicap, all cases have in common an impairment of the coordination of muscle action with an inability to maintain normal postures and balance and to perform normal movement and skills.

Clonus   alternate rapid muscle contraction and relaxation—indicative of central nervous system impairment.

Congenital   existing at, and usually before, birth.

Contraction   shortening of a muscle or ability of a muscle to develop tension.

Contracture   a fixed shortening of a muscle often causing restriction of joint motion.

Crossing the midline   the movement of the eyes, a hand and forearm, or foot and leg across the midsection of the body without involving any other part of the body, that is, without head turning, trunk twisting, or participation of the opposite limb.

Developmental disability   permanent impairment to an immature central nervous system that interferes with normal developmental processes in one or more areas; that is, speech language, adaptive behavior, gross motor skills, fine motor skills, and/or personal, socialization skills.

Developmental sequence   normal progression of motor skills including all areas such as fine motor, gross motor, personal, and social.

Dorsiflexion   upward motion of foot.

Dystocia   difficult labor.

Equilibrium reactions   brain mechanisms that function on a nonconscious level to preserve balance.

Equinus   refers to walking on toes.

Etiology   the study of the cause or sources of disease.

Extension   straightening of a joint or limb. In the *Extensor pattern,* the head and shoulders are arched back, the arms are straight, and the trunk is arched. In the severe extensor pattern, or *opisthotonus,* an extreme case would result in the heels touching the head.

Fine motor activities   activities or output in which precision of delicate muscle systems is required.

Flexion   bending of a joint or limb. In the *flexion pattern,* the head and shoulders are slumped forward, and the arms and legs bent.

Form perception   the ability to perceive an arrangement or pattern of elements or parts constituting a unitary whole.

Goniometer   instrument for measurement of joint range of motion (measures in units of degrees).

Gross motor activity   activities or output in which groups of large muscles are used and the factors of rhythm and balance are primary.

Hoyer lift   mechanical (hydraulic) device for lifting and transferring (heavy) individuals.

Hydrocephalus   excess fluid within the cranial cavity which may cause increased pressure on brain tissue, which may also cause an abnormally large head.

Hypertrophy   increase in bulk of tissue, especially muscle tissue.

IEP   individualized educational program. (See page 116 of text)

Integration   the pulling together and organizing of all the stimuli that are imposed on the organism at a given moment. It also involves the tying together with the present stimulation, experience variables retained from past activities, the organization of many individual movements into a complex response.

In utero   during the growth and development of the fetus in the uterus.

Kinesthetic the sense that yields knowledge of the muscles of the body and position of the joints.

Laterality complete motor awareness of the two sides of the body.

Long leg brace also called *K-A-F-O* orthotic device encompassing the knee and ankle joints; attaches to the shoe and extends up to the calf.

Long sitting sitting with legs extended straight out in front of body.

Lower extremities the legs.

Macrocephaly used to describe an abnormally large head.

Manual muscle test test of muscle strength through use of manual resistance.

Microcephaly used to describe an abnormally small head.

Midline imaginary line down the center of the body dividing left from right.

Motor test an objective method of determining the gross and fine motor abilities a child has at a given age. (Based on the chronological age at which a normal child acquires these motor skills.)

Muscle facilitation sensory input, manually or by apparatus, along with proper positioning, to encourage a muscle to work harder and in a more normal manner.

Muscle tone relates to the amount of tenseness in a muscle. The various degrees of tension are termed: *Spastic,* too much tone; *Athetoid,* hypotonic or too little tone with much involuntary motion; *Ataxic,* characterized by marked incoordination and disturbed equilibrium; *Rigid,* too much tone resulting in a "lead pipe" stiffness.

Opposition touching or pinching the pad of the thumb to the pad of the finger.

Orientation the child's ability to locate him or herself in space in relation to the things surrounding him or her in space and time. Also, the ability to stabilize his or her environment so that it remains more or less constant.

Palmar grasp   grasping an object in the palm of the hand using only fingers, not thumb.

Palmar surface   the palm of the hand.

Paralysis   loss or impairment of muscle function.

Perception   an experience or sensation combined or integrated with previous experiences which give it added meaning.

Perceptual-motor process   includes input (sensory or perceptual activities) and output (motor or muscular activities). The two cannot be divided because anything that happens to one area automatically affects the other.

Pincer grasp   grasping using thumb opposing a finger.

Plantar flexion   downward motion of foot.

Plantar surface   the sole of the foot.

Postural drainage   therapeutic drainage of lungs through proper positioning and percussion over the affected lung area.

Prehension   grasp.

Pronation   the position of the arm with palm downward.

Prone   lying on stomach.

Proprioception   sensory input from tissues of the body, for example, muscles and tendons, giving input about movements and position of the body.

Range of motion   (ROM) measurement of the amount of movement possible at joint.

Reciprocal motion   alternating movements of arms and legs; as in crawling, one hand moves first, the opposite knee is pulled up, the other hand is moved, followed by the opposite knee.

Righting reactions   mechanism within the brain that functions on a nonconscious basis to preserve alignment of head and body in relation to each other and to gravity.

Short leg brace   also called A-F-O; orthotic device encompassing the ankle joint; attaches to the shoe and extends up the calf.

Shunt   a device inserted in the cranial cavity to remove excess fluid, allowing it to drain into another body cavity, for example, the abdomen.

Side sitting sitting with knees bent and both knees facing in the same direction.

Sliding board rectangular board used to allow sliding transfers between bed and chair, chair and wheelchair, and so on.

Soft signs fine and gross motor incoordination or other abnormal movements believed to be related to perinatal complications.

Space perception the direct awareness of the spatial properties of an object, especially in relation to the observer, size, form, distance by any of the senses.

STNR (Symmetrical tonic neck reflex) flexing of head is accompanied by reflex flexing of arms and extension of legs. Extending head is accompanied with extending arms and flexing hips. Interferes with movement of upper and lower extremities, creeping, erect posture and looking down and working with hands.

Strabismus lack of coordination of the eye muscles so that the two eyes do not focus on the same point.

Subluxation partial dislocation or separation of a joint.

Supination the position of the arm with palm upward.

Supine lying flat on back.

Tactile pertaining to touch or touch pressure. *Tactile perception* is an ability to perceive tactile stimuli, as to localize, discriminate, qualify as in identification of form, shape, size, texture, and by touch pressure.

Tailor sitting sitting cross-legged on the floor, Indian style.

Therapeutic exercises exercises designed to improve or maintain muscle function.

Unilateral one-sided.

Upper extremities the arms.

Valgus foot turning outward; as when the foot is bent outward.

Varus foot turning inward; as when a person walks on the outer border of the foot.

WNL within normal limits.

References

Access Travel: Airports. Architectural and Transportation Barriers Compliance Board, Washington, DC.

Association of Retarded Citizens, Philadelphia Chapter. 1981. Prepare yourself. Bridge 1:15–16, 71.

Avery, M. E. 1978. New approaches to old problems in low birth weight infants. Research Report, p. 25. United Cerebral Palsy Research and Educational Foundation, New York.

Barsch, R. 1968. The Parent of the Handicapped Child. Charles C Thomas, Publisher, Springfield, IL.

Bax, M. C. 1964. Terminology and classifications of cerebral palsy. Dev. Med. Child Neurol. 6:259–297.

Bleck, E., and Nagel, D. A. (eds.). 1982. Physically Handicapped Children: A Medical Atlas for Teachers. 2nd Ed. Grune & Stratton, New York.

Block, J. D., and Silverstein, L. 1978. Integrating biofeedback/bioengineering approaches into a comprehensive cerebral palsy treatment center. Arch. Phys. Med. 59:525.

Bobath, B. 1967. The very early treatment of cerebral palsy. Dev. Med. Child Neurol. 9:373–390.

Bobath, B. 1973. The Concept of Neurodevelopmental Treatment. Western Cerebral Palsy Center, London.

Bobath, B., and Bobath, K. 1975. Motor Development in Different Types of Cerebral Palsy. William Heinemann Medical Books, Ltd., London.

Bobath, K. 1966. The Motor Deficits in Patients with Cerebral Palsy. Spastic International Medical Publications, Levenham, England.

Cardwell, V. 1956. Cerebral Palsy, Advances in Understanding and Care. Association for the Aid of Crippled Children, New York. p. 11.

Crothers, B., and Paine, R. 1959. The Natural History of Cerebral Palsy, p. 178. Harvard University Press, Cambridge, MA.

Cruikshank, W. M. (ed.). 1976. Cerebral Palsy, A Developmental Disability. Syracuse University Press, Syracuse, N.Y.

DeLellis, J. 1978. The Handicapped Driver's Mobility Guide. American Automobile Association, Falls Church, VA.

Donovan, B. 1978. The Cesarean Birth Experience. Beacon Press, Boston.

Downey, J., and Low, N. (eds.). 1974. The Child with Disabling Illness. Philadelphia, W. B. Saunders.

Driscoll, J. M., Driscoll, Y. T., Steir, M. E., Stark, R. I., Dangman, B. B., Perez, A., Wung, J. T., and Kritz, P. 1982. Mortality and morbidity in infants less than 1,001 grams birth weight. Pediatrics 60:21–25.

Ellenberg, J. H., and Nelson, K. B. 1981. Early recognition of infants at high risk for cerebral palsy: examination at age four months. Dev. Med. Child Neurol. 23:705–716.

Epilepsy Foundation of America. 1981a. Recognition and first aid for those with epilepsy. Washington, DC PI 15.

Epilepsy Foundation of America. 1981b. When surgery is an option. National Spokesman 14:5.

Finnie, N. 1975. Handling the Young Cerebral Palsied Child At Home. 2nd Ed. E. P. Dutton & Co., New York.

Fletcher, D., and Fredrick, J. 1981. Orthoses, ten steps for successful adjustment. Except. Parent 11:21–27.

Gilroy, J., and Meyer, J. S. 1979. Medical Neurology. Macmillan Publishing Co., New York.

Goldenson, R. (ed.). 1978. Disability and Rehabilitation Handbook. p. 332. McGraw-Hill, New York.

Green, A., and Mendelsohn, M. J. 1960. Is premedication necessary for handicapped children? J. Dent. Child. First quarter: 40–45.

Greene, J. W. 1978. Editorial comment. J. Obstet. Gynecol. 51:723.

Harris, M. M., and Dignam, P. F. 1980. A nonsurgical method of reducing drooling in cerebral palsied children. Dev. Med. Child Neurol. 22:293.

Haynes, U. 1979. A Developmental Approach to Casefinding. U.S. Department of Health and Human Services (Pub. 79-5210), p. 99. Washington, DC

Heppenstall, M. E., and Centerwall, W. R. 1977. An Introduction to Your Child Who Has Cerebral Palsy. Loma Linda University Press, Loma Linda, CA.

Holt, K. S. 1979. Medical examination of the child with cerebral palsy. Ped. Ann. 8:581–588.

Hughey, M. J., McElin, T. W., and Young, T. 1978. Maternal and fetal outcome of Lamaze-prepared patients. Obstet. Gynecol. J. 51:643–647.

International Society for Cerebral Palsy, Bulletin (London). 1981. Parents Issue, December: 21.

James, L. S., and Lanman, J. T. (eds.). 1976. Pediatrics 57 (Suppl., Part 2):635–642.

Joel, G. S. 1975. So Your Child Has Cerebral Palsy. p. 53. University of New Mexico Press, Albuquerque, NM.

Kaiser, I. H. 1979. A caution on amniocentesis, a letter to the editor. New York Times, Feb. 9, 1979.

Kew, S. 1975. Handicap and Family Crisis, Study of the Siblings of Handicapped Children. Pittman Publishing Co., London.

Kiely, J. L., Paneth, N., Stein, Z., and Susser, M. 1981. Cerebral palsy and newborn care. I. Secular trends in cerebral palsy. Dev. Med. Child Neurol. 23:537.

Krasner, P. R., and Silverstein, L. 1976. The preschool attainment record: A concurrent validity study with cerebral palsied children. Educ. Psychol. Movement 36:1049–1054.

Lee, C. L., and Bleck, E. E. 1980. Surgical correction of equinus deformity in cerebral palsy. Dev. Med. Child Neurol. 22:287–292.

Little, W. J. 1862. On the influence of Abnormal Parturition, Difficult Labours, Premature Birth, and Asphyxia Neonatorum, on the Mental and Physical Condition of the Child, Especially in Relation to Deformities. Transactions of the Obstetrical Society of London, Vol. III for the year 1861. Longman, Green, Longman, and Roberts, London.

Margulec, I. (ed.). 1966. Cerebral Palsy in Adolescence and Adulthood, Project No. O.V.R. 1-61, sponsored by Vocational Administration, Dept. H.E.W., USA and the American Joint Distribution Committee Services for Israel (Malben) Tel Aviv.

Mopsik, S. I., and Agard, J. A. (eds.). An Education Handbook for Parents of Handicapped Children. Abt Books, Cambridge, MA.

Neuwirth, R. 1980. Court rules that the disabled have the right to community services. UCP People, Nov./Dec.

New York State Education Department. 1980. Your Child's Right to an Education, A Guide for Parents of Handicapped Children in New York State. Albany, NY.

New York State Education Department. 1981. Newsbrief, Vol. IV No. 4. Office for the Education of Children with Handicapping Conditions, Albany, NY.

Office of Information, Resources for the Handicapped. 1981. Programs for the Handicapped. Department of Health and Human Services, Washington, DC.

O'Reilly, D. E., and Walentynowicz, J. E. 1981. Etiological factors in cerebral palsy: An historical review. Dev. Med. Child Neurol. 23:635.

Paneth, N., Kiely, J., Stein, Z., and Susser, M. 1981. Cerebral palsy and newborn care. Dev. Med. Child Neurol. 23:806.

Paneth, N., Kiely, J., Stein, Z., and Susser, M. 1981. The incidence of cerebral palsy: which way are we going? Dev. Med. Child Neurol. 23:111.

Phelps, W. M. 1950. Etiology and diagnostic classification of cerebral palsy. In: Proceedings of the Cerebral Palsy Institute. Association for Aid of Crippled Children, New York.

The President's Committee on Employment of the Handicapped. 1981. Affirmative Action to Employ Handicapped People. Washington, DC.

Rauth, M. 1980. Mainstreaming, A River to Nowhere or a Promising Current? American Federation of Teachers, Washington, DC.

Rauth, M. 1981. The Education for All Handicapped Children Act (P.L. 94-142). Preserving Both Children's and Teachers' Rights. American Federation of Teachers, AFL-CIO, Washington, DC.

Richmond, J. B. 1978. Investing in Our Children. Research Report, p. 14. United Cerebral Palsy Research and Educational Foundation, New York.

Rinsky, L. A., and Kleinman, R. G. 1981. Surgical treatment of scoliosis in cerebral palsy. Bulletin 101, Vol. 32 No. 1. American Academy for Cerebral Palsy and Developmental Medicine Bulletin, Richmond, VA.

Robert Woods Foundation. 1979. Dental Care for Handicapped Americans. Special Report No. 2. Robert Woods Foundation, Princeton, NJ.

Robinault, I. 1973. Functional Aids for the Multiply Handicapped. Harper Row, Publisher, New York.

Rosenstein, S. 1978. Dentistry in Cerebral Palsy and Related Handicapping Conditions. Charles C Thomas, Springfield, IL.

Rothman, J. G. 1978. Effects of respiratory exercises on vital capacity and forced expiratory volume in children with cerebral palsy. Phys. Ther. 58:421.

Rusk, H. 1977. Rehabilitation Medicine, Fourth Edition. C. V. Mosby, St. Louis., p. 477.

Scherzer, A. L. 1974. Early diagnosis, treatment and management of cerebral palsy. In Rehabilitation Literature. National Society for Crippled Children and Adults, Chicago.

Scherzer, A. L., and Mike, V. 1974. Cerebral palsy and the low birth weight child. Am. J. Disord. Child. 128:199–203.

Schleichkorn, J. 1980. Informational needs of parents of children with cerebral palsy. Unpublished report, The Union for Experimenting Colleges and Universities, Cincinnati, OH.

Schleichkorn, J., and Manus, M. 1971. Study of Adults with Cerebral Palsy. United Cerebral Palsy Associations, New York.

Schlesinger, E. R., Allaway, N. C., and Petlin, S. 1959. Survivorship in cerebral palsy. Am. J. Public Health 40:343–349.

Seliger, S. 1981. The modern woman's guide to having a healthy baby. Washingtonian 16:76–81.

Stembera, Z., Anamenacek, K., and Polacek, K. 1976. High Risk Pregnancy and Child. Martnus/Mijhoff/Medical Division, The Hague.

Sternfeld, L. 1978. Report of the Medical Director. United Cerebral Palsy Research and Educational Foundation, Annual Report, No. 6, New York.

Thompson, R. J., and O'Quinn, A. N. 1979. Developmental Disabilities, p. 136. Oxford University Press, New York.

United Nations. 1976. Obstacles Limiting Access of Disabled Children to Rehabilitation Services. Report ST/ESA/47. p. 13. New York.

Velleman, R. 1979. Serving Physically Disabled People, pp. 371–372. R. W. Bowker, New York.

Warfel, J. H., and Schlagenhauff, R. E. 1980. Understanding Neurologic Diseases. Urban and Schwarzenberg, Publishers, Baltimore.

Warren, R. D., and Dickman, I. R. 1981. For This Respite, Much Thanks, p. 3. United Cerebral Palsy Associations, New York.

Wegman, M. 1981. Annual summary of vital statistics—1980. Pediatrics 68(6):755.

Recommended Reading

Ambrom, S. 1975. Child Development. Rinehart Press, San Francisco.

Berkow, R. (ed.). 1977. The Merck Manual. Merck, Sharpe and Dohme, Publishers, Rahway, NJ.

Black, J. 1972. Neonatal Emergencies and Other Problems. Appleton-Crofts, Publishers, New York.

Bobath, B., and Finnie, N. 1970. Problems of communication between parents and staff in the treatment and management of children with cerebral palsy. Dev. Med. Child Neurol. 12:629–635.

Bowe, F. 1978. Handicapping America, Barriers to Disabled People. Harper and Row, New York.

Brown, M. S. 1979. How to tell if a baby has cerebral palsy and what to tell his parents when he does. Nursing '79 May:88–93.

Bruck, L. 1978. Access, The Guide to Better Life for Disabled Americans. David Obst Books. Random House, New York.

Chalfant, J., and Van Dusen Pysh, M. 1980. The Compliance Manual. Pem Press, New Rochelle, NY.

Clelland, C. C. 1978. Mental Retardation, A Developmental Approach. Prentice-Hall, Inc. Englewood Cliffs, NJ.

Denhoff, E. 1967. Cerebral Palsy—The Preschool Years. Charles C Thomas, Springfield, IL.

Drillien, C. M. 1958. Growth and development in a group of children with very low birth weight. J. Disabl. Child. 33:10–18.

Featherstone, H. 1980. A Difference in the Family—Life with a Disabled Child. Basic Books, Inc., New York.

Freeman, R. D. 1967. Controversy over patterning as a treatment for brain damaged children. JAMA 202:385–388.

Gesell, A., and Ilg, F. L. 1949. Child Development. Harper, New York.

Heslinga, K. 1974. Not Made of Stone—The Sexual Problems of Handicapped People. Charles C Thomas, Springfield, IL.

Humebaugh, A. (ed.). 1978. Directory for Exceptional Children. Porter-Sargent Publishers, Boston.

JAMA (Journal of the American Medical Association). 1978. Brain stimulation for seizures, spasticity needs better evaluation. June.

Keats, S. 1975. Cerebral Palsy. Charles C Thomas, Springfield, IL.

Levitt, S. 1977. Treatment of Cerebral Palsy and Motor Delay. Blackwell Scientific Publications, London.

McDonald, E. T., and Chance, B. 1964. Cerebral Palsy. Prentice-Hall, Inc., Englewood Cliffs, NJ.

Pearlman, L., and Scott, K. A. 1981. Raising the Handicapped Child. Prentice-Hall, Inc., Englewood Cliffs, NJ.

Rafael, B. 1977. Enlarging the circle, the parent infant program at United Cerebral Palsy of New York City. Teach. Except. Child. Spring.

Ryan, S. A., and Clayton, B. D. 1981. Handbook of Practical Pharmacology. C. V. Mosby, St. Louis, MO.

Salter, R. B. 1970. Textbook of Disorders and Injuries of the Musculoskeletal System. Williams & Wilkins, Baltimore.

Silverman, H. 1980. Communication for the Speechless, Prentice-Hall, Inc. Englewood Cliffs, NJ.

Surburg, P. R. 1981. Implications of Public Law 94-142 for physical therapists. Phys. Ther. 61:210–212.

Tibbits, D. 1980. A Guide to Survival for Disabled Students. Office of the Disabled, State University of New York at Stony Brook.

UCPeople. Newsletter of the United Cerebral Palsy Associations, Inc. published bimonthly, New York.

U.S. Department of Health and Human Services. 1979. Pocket Guide to Federal Help for Disabled Persons. Office of Information and Resources for the Handicapped, Washington, DC.